Behavioral Medicine

Health care costs and the effective management of health care are of primary importance and concern to federal, state, and local governments. Consequently, it is necessary to develop innovative, successful, and integrated cost-effective treatments and procedures. *Behavioral Medicine* presents a new model to address these needs.

Behavioral Medicine discusses the composition of effective psychosocial treatment and presents a cost analysis of social work and its services. By defining the problems that need to be addressed in health care costs and management, applying research, and using studies, this text presents an effective model for health care organizations. It also presents a profile of the behavioral social worker, which defines the abilities needed to be effective in the role and looks at the key impact areas for a behavioral health model. This is a comprehensive guide for social workers preparing to work in health care organizations, and for existing social workers, academics, and practitioners of behavioral medicine in health settings.

John S. Wodarski is Professor at the College of Social Work, University of Tennessee.

D1475222

Behavioral Medicine
A Social Worker's Guide

John S. Wodarski

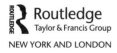

Routledge
Taylor & Francis Group

NEW YORK AND LONDON

First published 2009
by Routledge
270 Madison Ave, New York, NY 10016

Simultaneously published in the UK
by Routledge
2 Park Square, Milton Park, Abingdon, Oxon OX14 4RN

Routledge is an imprint of the Taylor & Francis Group, an informa business

© 2009 Taylor & Francis

Typeset in Galliard by
Florence Production Ltd, Stoodleigh, Devon
Printed and bound in the United States of America on acid-free paper by
Edwards Brothers, Inc.

Library of Congress Cataloging-in-Publication Data
Wodarski, John S.
   Behavioral medicine: a social worker's guide/John S. Wodarski.
      p. cm.
      Includes bibliographical references.
   1. Medicine and psychology.   I. Title.
   1. Behavioral Medicine—organization & administration.   2. Social
   Work—organization & administration.   3. Behavioral Medicine—methods.
   4. Social Work—methods.
   R726.5.W63 2008
   616.001'9—dc22   2008026703

ISBN10: 0–7890–2519–1 (hbk)
ISBN10: 0–7890–2916–2 (pbk)
ISBN10: 0–203–88491–4 (ebk)

ISBN13: 978–0–7890–2519–7 (hbk)
ISBN13: 978–0–7890–2916–4 (pbk)
ISBN13: 978–0–203–88491–1 (ebk)

Contents

Preface

Amid changes in the health care industry will come changes to managed health care as it is now known. This book focuses on three paradigm shifts presently taking place: the effectiveness of health care, the cost efficiency of health care systems, and the service integration of fragmented systems; specifically those of health and mental health (Law, 2006; Munsey, 2006; Wodarski, 2000).

Increased costs and proposed budget cuts are forcing segregated systems into an overall integrated system of delivery (Meyers, 2006). The model proposed here, "The Integrated Human Service Delivery System: A Human Service Model," employs a change in the policies and procedures that are presently at work in human service systems. The model suggests a progressive approach to service integration through a case management modality. This modality suggests that the Behavioral Health Social Worker (BHSW) case manager will supervise and control services provided for each client or case. The model provides a cost-effective delivery system that will provide the needed psychosocial treatment, currently at risk of becoming fragmented as health care programs are revamped.

In addition to routine health care needs, the majority of patients receiving services through their health care provider also suffer from psychological and psychosocial problems. In fact, researchers have found "that between 30 percent and 80 percent (depending on the study) of all primary care visits are driven in significant part by behavioral health issues" (Schaible et al., 2004). As these patients typically will only receive medical services from their primary care physician (PCP), they most likely will not receive the psychosocial treatment necessary for overall health. Historically, psychosocial treatment would have been provided exclusively by social work professionals employed through social service agencies. This separation of care causes a major deficit in the collective health of our nation, as most health authorities now believe that major improvements could be affected through lifestyle changes. In fact, certain research indicates that psychosocial variables contribute as much as 70 percent of the variance of chronic diseases (Leukefeld, 1989; Matthews, 2005; Packard, 2005). Research has also shown that "each illness type has its own specific psychosocial problems, more or less unique stressors that usually emerge with considerable clarity from the constellation of symptoms of a particular illness and the special conditions that characterize its management and treatment" (Cummings, 1992). One could conclude that an emphasis on remedial and preventative health care—now averaging one billion dollars a day—will result in an increased need for health care practitioners trained in behavioral medicine (Stoesz, 1986; Ugland, 1989).

In January 2000, the U.S. Surgeon General, Dr. David Satcher issued the first-ever "Surgeon General's Report on Mental Health." His stated intent was to alert the "American people that mental illness is a critical public health problem that must be addressed immediately" (Satcher, 2000). Dr. Satcher notes that many mental and behavioral illnesses go untreated as a result of the stigma attached to mental disease, and the "lack of parity between insurance coverage for mental health services and other health care services." The bulk of the Surgeon General's report is dedicated to his vision for the future and recommendations to overcome the aforementioned barriers. Included in his recommendations are the following points that relate directly to the needed marriage of basic health care and mental health treatment:

- Improve Public Awareness of Effective Treatments
- Ensure the Supply of Mental Health Services and Providers
- Ensure Delivery of State-of-the-Art Treatments

  - Ensure that mental health services are as universally accessible as other health services in the continuously changing health care delivery system.

- Tailor Treatment to Individuals, Acknowledging Age, Gender, Race, and Culture
- Facilitate Entry into Treatment

  - Ensure ready access to appropriate services for people ... to significantly reduce the need for involuntary care, which is sometimes required in order to prevent behavior that could be harmful

- Reduce Financial Barriers to Treatment

(Satcher, 2000)

In addition to the basic need to improve availability and affordability of mental health care services, most major health problems facing our nation involve psychological causes, correlates, or consequences. Training in behavioral medicine and interventions, along with competency in assessing psychosocial factors, is therefore a must and should occupy a central position in all levels of education. Solutions and prevention require changes in attitudes, values, behavior, and lifestyles. A few basic examples are:

- AIDS and other sexually transmitted diseases with controllable risk factors.
- Addictive processes in substance abuse and other self-destructive practices.
- Obesity-related morbidity, such as diabetes and heart disease.
- Stress at work and at home that weakens the immune system.

Although it is apparent that behavioral health care interventions are beneficial to the nation, state and local governments continue to cut back on prevention programs. These cutbacks are due primarily to the changing structure of health care and the exponential increase in its cost. Instead of actually decreasing overall cost, however, these initial attempts to reduce preventative measures will actually result in cost ineffectiveness.

This text outlines the composition of effective psychosocial treatment and presents a cost analysis of social work and its services. It also presents a profile of the Behavioral Health Social Worker (BHSW), which defines the abilities of an effective behavioral social worker. Among the attributes required, are: (1) the depth of an acceptable knowledge base; (2) the behavioral skills necessary for an intellectual and conceptual understanding of theories of human development and learning; and (3) the utilization of techniques necessary to bring about behavioral changes in clinical practice. A foundation for the emerging roles of behavioral interventions in primary care is formed from these characteristics. In addition, the key impact areas for a behavioral health model are delineated. The behavioral interventions provided by the BHSW will ultimately increase the quality of psychosocial health care, while simultaneously controlling medical costs.

Health care costs and the effective management of health care are of primary importance and concern to federal, state, and local governments. Consequently, it is necessary to develop innovative, successful, and integrated cost-effective treatments and procedures. This text proposes such procedures by defining the problems to be addressed, applying research and studies for support, and presenting an innovative model for cost-effective managed health care combined with empirically based psychosocial intervention and prevention.

Abbreviations

BHSW	Behavioral Health Social Worker
BMI	Body Mass Index
BSW	Bachelor of Social Work
CDC	Center for Disease Control and Prevention
CPR	Center for Prevention Research
DAPA	Diagnostic Assessment for Physical Ailments
FASI	Family Assessment Service Integrity
GAPS	Guidelines for Adolescents Preventive Services
GHQ	General Health Questionnaire
GSI	Global Screening Inventory
HMO	Health Management Organization
IOM	Institute of Medicine
IVSET	Interactive Videodisc for Special Education Technology
LSTIM	Life Skills Training Information Model
MAAS	Multidimensional Adolescent Assessment Scale
MAST	Michigan Alcoholism Screening Test
MMPI	Minnesota Multiphasic Personality Inventory
MPSI	Multi-Problem Screening Industry
MSSW	Master of Science in Social Work
MSW	Master of Social Work
NASW	National Association of Social Workers
NCSPAS	National Computer Systems Professional Assessment Service
NIMH	National Institute of Mental Health
OAPP	Office of Adolescent Pregnancy Programs
PCP	primary care physician
RAI	rapid assessment instrument
SPR	Society for Prevention Research
TGT	Teams–Games–Tournaments
WIC	Women, Infants and Children's Programs
WOR	Ways of Responding

1 Behavioral Medicine and Managed Care

Implications for Social Work Practice*

Historically in American health care, the physician has assumed primary responsibility for an individual's care during times of illness. The patient passively awaits the doctor's judgment, perhaps in anticipation of an instantaneous cure. The healthy individual, on the other hand, generally takes his/her physiological state for granted. This reliance on the family physician as primary change agent was reasonable and necessary prior to the 1960s, considering that infectious diseases were the number one health problem in the U.S. (Sultz & Young, 1997; Wodarski et al., 1991). At the dawn of the age of antibiotics, however, the public health burden shifted to those chronic diseases that have been related to unhealthy lifestyle choices. In fact, according to the Center for Disease Control, the top ten leading causes of death, up to 70 percent, are related to lifestyle or preventable illnesses (Rains & Erickson, 1997). In conjunction with this shift, the illness industry has seen major growth in the United States. Health care expenditures account for nearly 16 percent of the gross domestic product (Sultz & Young, 1997), while federal and state service programs grew 1,760 percent, or 32.3 billion dollars, from 1960 to 1985 (el-Askari et al., 1998); however, even with this increased funding, many public health problems have continued to increase. Health costs are rising 1 percent annually.

By improving health and quality of life, many agree that a significant reduction in health care cost could be achieved through the prevention of chronic illness. The role that prevention will play in the light of managed care is unclear, as the standard approach to human services places an emphasis on the deficiencies of the individual (el-Askari et al., 1998). This approach undermines a client's self-worth in addition to decreasing a sense of responsibility for his or her own well being. Although this is an unintended effect of human services programs, it is also a very significant one. Literature suggests that there is a strong association between disempowerment (a lack of social support and weak community involvement) and poor health. Therefore, the traditional approach to health care programs may be contributing to the poor health of individuals by identifying the problems and attempting to ameliorate them (el-Askari et al., 1998).

* Chapter written with the assistance of: Amber Brauckmuller, Stephanie Swain, and Michael Waltke.

Key among trends in behavioral medicine is a "growing demand for and use of integrated, comprehensive health services that blend health and behavior, prevention, health promotion, and disease management" (Clay, 2005; Kersting, 2005a). The new field of behavioral medicine seeks to broaden health care to include active client responsibility in the treatment of disease and the maintenance of health. The emphasis is on the alteration of maladaptive behavior patterns that constitute an unhealthy lifestyle (Jeffery, 1989). Success with behavioral strategies in the treatment of various mental disorders paved the way to the later application of these powerful technologies to medically related problems, such as stress disorders and obesity (Thyer & Wodarski, 1998; Wodarski & Wodarski, 2004). These intervention procedures with proven successful histories have encouraged the wider acceptance of behavioral treatments by the empirically oriented medical community (Agras, 1982; Blanchard, 1982; Eysenck, 1988; Krantz & Blumethal, 1987; Pinkerton et al., 1982; Pomerleau, 1982).

This chapter reviews the behavioral medicine paradigm and its implications relevant to social work practice in health care settings. It also focuses on the role of the social worker in the application of behavioral techniques in managed health care settings and elaborates requisite practice principles.

Managed Care and Behavioral Health

Monumental economic and political forces are in the process of reshaping the way health and mental health services will be delivered in the United States. Managed care is simply a harbinger of this fundamental paradigm shift, which will involve the re-engineering of health care in general in terms of effectiveness, cost, and integration (Cummings, 1995; Kent & Hersen, 2000; Strosahl, 1994, 1995). Not only will there be an unrelenting focus on developing cost efficient delivery systems, but the watchword in the next generation of health care will be service integration and effectiveness. Formerly segregated delivery systems, for example, health and mental health, will be pressured to merge because of growing popularity of capitation, the preferred model for financing health care, and the realization that psychosocial variables impact physical health. "Implementation of managed care principles in the mental health arena has generated much debate, particularly with respect to issues of quality of care" (Sanchez & Turner 2003). As noted by Dr. David Barlow, "in an era of evidence-based practice, psychological treatments have been shown to be the equal of or to be superior to alternative medical or pharmacological treatments" (Kersting, 2005b). The arbitrary division of mind and body will give way to the stark financial reality that health care costs cannot be contained as long as physical health and mental health care are structured as non-overlapping enterprises.

Although managed care is likely to ratchet down the cost of specific medical and mental health procedures, there will be no way to coordinate the utilization of services without integrating the two systems. In other words, such a great proportion of medical care is driven by psychological and psychosocial concerns that the ability of the two systems to contain utilization and cost depends on the provision of appropriate behavioral health services in the general medical setting (Friedman et al., 1995).

The *de facto* mental health system in the United States is primary medical care (Rieger et al., 1993). This ascendancy of the primary care physician as the major provider of behavioral health services is most likely the result of three developments in the field of mental health: (a) the introduction of selective serotonin reuptake inhibitors (SSRIs); (b) the failure of behavioral health carve outs to meet the needs of mental health consumers; and (c) the increasing recognition of the benefits found in an integrated system of medical and behavioral care (Gray et al., 2005).

The provider constituency in primary care includes a rather bewildering number of physicians (e.g. family practice, general internal medicine, obstetrics-gynecology, pediatrics) and allied health care groups (e.g. physician's assistants, clinical nurse specialists, registered and licensed nurses, women's health care specialist), all of whom are providing routine medical care and are likely to encounter patients with mental disorders or significant psychosocial stresses. Enrollment in managed care plans (e.g., HMOs) has increased dramatically. In 1973 approximately 5 million people participated in these programs, whereas in 1992 the number was an estimated 100 million (MacLeod, 1995), and in 1997 approximately 160 million were enrolled (Callister & Wall, 2001; Findlay, 1998). Indeed, research indicates that half of all informal mental health care in the United States is delivered solely by the above-mentioned providers (Narrow et al., 1993). Other data gathered on this topic states that approximately "60 percent of all mental health care visits related to mental health are to primary care physicians" (Pace et al., 1995). Factors that may have a great influence on this trend of seeking primary care physicians as the sole mental health provider include easier access, confidentiality concerns, social definitions, and public perception/stigmatization of the utilization of mental health services (Pace et al., 1995).

Interestingly, nearly half of all individuals with a diagnosable mental disorder seek no mental health care from any professional, but 80 percent of these individuals will visit their primary care physician at least yearly. Visits are usually very short and of diagnostic nature. For many patients with psychological or psychosocial concerns, medical visits are generated by the physical symptoms of distress (Smith et al., 1995). For example, a recent study of the ten most common physical complaints in primary care revealed that 85 percent end up with no diagnosable organic etiology during a three-year follow-up period (Kroenke & Mangelsdorf, 1989).

Managed Care, Assessment Instruments, and Helping Professionals

The stringent standards required by managed health care have changed the way that service is delivered by all human service agencies. The managed care system now requires helping professionals (physicians, psychologists, social workers, etc.) to be accountable for the types of service they provide, the type of clientele that they serve, and the expense, duration, and outcome of the services provided. Part of being an accountable practitioner is working from an empirical basis in relation to interventions, data collection, and treatment process (Wodarski, 1997). This emphasis on accountability comes in response to the decreasing federal and state monetary and philosophical support (Wodarski, 1997). Therefore, professionals are required to work accurately, swiftly, empirically, and in limited amount of time, while delivering services that are ever more effective and cost-efficient.

Levels of involvement in managed care appeared to increase from 1996 to 2001, but ratings of specific stresses associated with managed care, such as external constraints on services, managed care paperwork, managed care reimbursements rates, and excessive paperwork, did not increase, nor did sources of satisfaction (Baird & Rupert, 2004). The standardized requirements of managed care have turned the profession toward recreating rapid assessment instruments (RAI) that are easy to administer, score, and complete without losing validity or reliability.

Many instruments exist that are reliable and valid when measuring one aspect of a problem or a particular diagnosis; however, the need is growing for an instrument that can provide the worker with a differential diagnosis for problems related to substance abuse or physical/mental health concerns. This instrument will assist the professional in creating a quicker, more accurate assessment of problems, so that they can refer clients to the appropriate helping agent. RAIs also highlight what areas might have compounded, as well as contributing factors, which often remain unnoticed when helping professionals zero in on their own area of expertise. This approach requires a more collaborative and interactive component on the part of helping professionals. There is no reason to doubt that RAIs combined with the interdisciplinary team approach can be an effective way to navigate through managed care systems (Resnick & Tighe, 1997).

The goal of managed care is to alter the treatment process in hopes of reducing the amount of unnecessary health service utilization (Berkman, 1996). The treatment process currently experiences budget, service integration, and utilization constraints. There are financial rewards for service providers who limit services, and pre-establishing treatment plan/goals with regular reviews are becoming the norm (Wodarski et al., 2001). The more powerful role of managed care organizations has also impacted the decision making process regarding which services will be provided. In the past, exclusively physicians and clients made these decisions; however, the managed care organization is now the primary decision maker (Raw, 1999).

Rapid Assessment

Rapid assessment techniques have become increasingly popular with practitioners and agencies alike. The trend in using rapid assessment techniques has been associated with the recent demand by funding agencies for evidence that clients are reaching their stated goals and that programs are effective in treating their clients. Both practitioners and agencies have realized the contribution of rapid assessment instruments in meeting these two aims. In the managed care arena, there is no doubt that rapid assessment technology would be welcomed.

Social workers who work with children, adults, and multi-problem families, need to assess multiple sources of data across and beyond family systems. At the present time, many professionals use clinical interviews, personal judgment, and assumptions to make decisions about services and treatment needs. The danger in this is clear. By utilizing RAI techniques, the Bachelor of Social Work (BSW) can readily assess problems that may impact the individual patient's physical health. The patient would be assessed for alcohol and drug problems, mental illness, family violence, child abuse, housing needs, depression, nutrition, financial problems, etc. This information would then be utilized to provide the patient with an integrated individualized treatment plan and appropriate referrals. By utilizing these valid assessments, the social worker increases his/her chance of making an accurate evaluation of all the psychosocial needs that may be impacting the patient's physical health. No area would be left out, thus making the use of these instruments much more efficient and effective than personal judgment. With appropriate, accurate assessment, the patient would receive only the referrals/services that were indicated.

The information gathered from the rapid assessment instruments would not necessarily be used solely for the primary care physician. Rather, this information with client consent could be forwarded to the service agencies where the client would be referred for further treatment. This process would assist the service agencies by providing reliable information about the client's problems prior to the first meeting. It would also reduce replicated information gathering by the service agencies. Again, efficiency and integration would be increased, thereby decreasing the cost. Two necessary objectives for RAIs are the ability to accurately assess clients' needs and to evaluate the effectiveness of program interventions.

Social workers have begun to identify the utility of RAIs to collect large quantities of data of high quality. Studies have consistently found that these instruments are easily administered, cost-effective, and can provide reliable client data (McMahon, 1984; Rapp-Paglicci et al., 2000; Streever et al.,

1984). In addition, these assessment instruments are more objective than a personal interview, in that the personal biases of the worker are reduced, and the subjective nature of assessment, as a whole, is decreased. Flowers et al. (1993) found that clients who were given RAIs throughout treatment made more improvement on their goals, terminated from treatment less often, and were in general more satisfied with treatment. These instruments have also been noted to gather more information from clients in a shorter amount of time. Consequently, these instruments are more efficient as well as more accurate.

Social workers who work with lifestyle behaviors leading to problematic health must assess multiple sources of data across and beyond family systems. For social workers who work with substance abuse clients, the need for accurate and reliable information is critical because of the serious decisions that must be made for effective intervention to take place (Thyer & Wodarski, 1998).

RAI Model for Differential Diagnosis

The top three RAIs found effective for assessing difficulties in the fields of alcohol abuse, mental health, and physical health, are CAGE, the GHQ-12 or GSI-25, and DAPA. All of these scales can be implemented in a primary care setting and can yield rapid and accurate assessments, allowing for appropriate referrals to a worker on the team in a corresponding discipline. In addition, these instruments can be administered with ease, are simple to score, and are supported by empirical evidence of their validity and reliability. Their use is extensively discussed in Chapter Four.

Numerous findings reveal that primary care physicians often overlook significant mental disorders (Berwick et al., 1991) and alcohol abuse in their patients (Lairson et al., 1992). Liskow et al. (1995) have found that an average of 20–30 percent of clients in clinical settings have alcohol related problems, and that out of this 20–30 percent, physicians only detect between 10 and 50 percent of those afflicted. Of the patients with mental disorders, half or more go undiagnosed and untreated (Berwick et al., 1991). As a result, many of the presenting problems that patients are being treated for may be compounded by mental health and alcohol complications. It is apparent that the utilization of RAIs on the dual diagnosis population would also be beneficial.

Interdisciplinary Team Model

"Collaborative care can and should take place at all levels of health care . . . Outpatient, inpatient, long-term, emergency, pediatrics, it fits in everywhere" says Dr. Margaret Heldring (Kersting, 2005b: 57). The idea of using an interdisciplinary team approach to provide appropriate client care has become widespread (Resnick & Tighe, 1997). The interdisciplinary team generally contains social workers, physicians, physician assistants, psychiatrists, and other paraprofessionals. Utilizing this model leads to more accurate diagnoses, more efficient use of a professional's time, a decrease in cost, and more appropriate client care (Resnick & Tighe, 1997). The interdisciplinary team approach requires that members of the team interact within their area of expertise, maximizing the use of their education. The enhanced function of the role differentiation in this model enables professionals to meet the needs of a greater number of clients at a lower cost (Resnick & Tighe, 1997). The cost reductions involved in the utilization of this model allow managed care companies to expand their scope in a greater attempt to achieve nationwide health care.

> Unless the complex social and medical needs of patients are recognized and unless a comprehensive package of services is provided based on an interdisciplinary health care model (including social workers), a majority of Americans will be under insured or forced to pay significant additional fees for uncovered service or supplemental insurance.
>
> (Mizrahi, 1993, p. 89)

Benefits

Despite the role changes for social workers created by managed care, social workers' expertise and experience is still essential to social work practice. It has been found that 20–80 percent of primary care visits result in the medication of presenting problems that are frequently of psychological origin (Resnick & Tighe, 1997). As a result, the strain on physicians' time for non-medical problems is inordinate (Resnick & Tighe, 1997). With social workers performing the initial assessments of client needs through RAIs, the entire interdisciplinary team will benefit. Social workers will assess and refer, as is appropriate, to other more appropriate providers, allowing physicians more time to deal with medical problems. Social workers also have the ability to flag the psychosocial aspects of ailments, again saving the physician the time needed to screen the client/patient (Resnick & Tighe, 1997). In addition, the social workers can reveal information about a client's psychological problems, which will enable the physician to deliver more comprehensive patient care (Berkman, 1996). Besides helping the physician to address the mental health needs of the client, social workers can also work within the primary care setting to address the client's environmental, psychological, and financial concerns. Social workers can work with clients on family issues, financial and resource concerns, mental health issues, behavioral problems, medical noncompliance, etc. (Gross et al., 1983). The assisting role of the social worker allows for service delivery to run smoothly, appropriately, and effectively.

The inclusion of the role of a social worker as a member of the inter-disciplinary team can also yield financial rewards to physicians, insurance providers, and other professionals on the team. Collaboration between the medical/behavioral health providers has helped to identify optimal billing agents and improved reimbursement rates. Schaible et al. (2004) found that third-party payment for out-patient mental health services increased by 500 percent in 4 years, replacing state funding as the largest source of payment for outpatient mental health treatment in a pilot program that integrated medical/behavioral health treatment. The preventive measures utilized by social workers reduces costs through early detection, early intervention, and decreased use/re-use of hospital services (Berkman, 1996). Potential savings can be achieved through billing on a fee-for-service basis, seeking grants, and consultations (Hookey, 1979). Social workers will also benefit from the time constraints required by managed care in that they will be able to serve a greater number of clients in an allotted amount of time, and they are less likely to experience the amount of burnout and replacement that is currently threatening the profession.

Including the social workers as members of an interdisciplinary team offers financial incentives for the primary care physicians (Berkman, 1996).

> Medicare considers each patient visit as potentially billable, so a physician can free up valuable billable hours when the social worker has relieved the doctor of the need to spend time providing attention and arranging home care services, family meetings, and the like.
>
> (Berkman, 1996, p. 545)

In addition to financially serving physicians, the interdisciplinary team approach using RAIs reduces the strain on medical staff, which enables them to serve more patients/clients at lower rates (Resnick & Tighe, 1997).

Managed care companies and other insurance agents also stand to benefit from the utilization of social workers as part of the interdisciplinary team. The early detection and intervention of mental health problems by social workers significantly reduces the potential cost of treatment. Research has also found that early detection of mental health problems reduces the likelihood that patients will seek medical attention for psychological problems (Berkman, 1996).

Social Learning Techniques: The Foundation for Behavioral Medicine

One aspect of the service provided by the professional behavioral health social worker includes the application of social learning techniques, which are being used increasingly in the field of preventative medicine. Medical research has accumulated overwhelming evidence that identifies specific lifestyle factors that place an individual at risk for the development of specific types of diseases. Breslow and Enstrom (1980) summarize this evidence to isolate seven health practices that extend life:

1   Never smoke cigarettes.
2   Get regular physical activity.
3   Use alcohol moderately or not at all.
4   Get 7 to 8 hours of sleep per night.
5   Maintain proper weight.
6   Eat breakfast.
7   Do not eat between meals.

Social learning techniques can be used to initiate and maintain these practices, thus reducing risk factors and preventing the disease's development. Taylor (1999) proposes that because chronic illness has become our major health problem, its physical, vocational, social, and psychological consequences . . . are of increasing significance and indicate the need for behavioral health interventions that work in concert with primary care (Taylor, 1999). Moreover, social learning techniques may be used in the prevention of any disease for which lifestyle risk factors have been identified (Abeles, 1986; Dingfelder, 2006).

Perhaps the most important factor contributing to a successful social learning therapy strategy is a complete and individualized assessment of the problem behaviors. The assessment not only specifies the target problem, but also indicates the conditions that constitute a resolution of the problem. Pinkerton and Associates (1982) suggest four steps for a comprehensive behavioral assessment.

1. In observable terms, define the target behavior.
2. Specify the antecedent events that elicit or precipitate the problem behavior, and the consequences that maintain the behavior.
3. Quantify the target behavior and related variables in terms of rate, frequency, and duration of occurrence.
4. Specify in quantitative terms the desired goal or outcome.

Self-monitoring is a frequently used behavior assessment method, as it involves the client's observation and systematic recording of behaviors and their antecedents and consequences. This strategy forces the client to become very aware of the behavior, which in itself often facilitates a certain degree of behavior change. The process renders data that is also quite useful in the evaluation of treatment effectiveness (Cincirpini & Floreen, 1982; Stuart, 1967; Thyer & Wodarski, 1998).

Treatment Options Relevant to Social Learning Techniques

Inasmuch as environmental factors play an important role in today's illnesses, the basic learning techniques of respondent and operant conditioning, which operate on environmental influences, are choice treatments in behavioral medicine (Pinkerton et al., 1982). The basic techniques of social learning theory are grounded in the conditioning theories, which essentially state that learning occurs through prior experiences, and that behavior is usually influenced by its consequences (Bandura, 1977). Departing from the traditional socio-behavioral view, in which behavior is merely controlled by external consequences, it has become clear to social learning theorists that cognitive variables, that is, one's expectations about the ability of self-change, come in to play in the mediation of behavior (Wodarski, 1985; Wodarski & Dziegielewski, 2002). Consequently, cognitive strategies are now integrated with most behavioral medicine strategies. Also incorporated into this schema are principles showing that learning that occurs through direct experience can also occur through the observation of others (modeling) (Bandura, 1977).

Respondent Techniques

Respondent behaviors are those that are considered to be elicited by preceding stimuli and involve an involuntary response or "reflex." These would include the salivation response to food or an increased heart rate in response to social stress. Because emotional behavior is generally elicited by preceding stimuli, it is frequently classified as respondent behavior as well (Pinkerton et al., 1982). Respondent conditioning, then, occurs when after repeated pairings a neutral stimulus acquires the eliciting properties of the original stimulus.

Relaxation therapy (meditation) is a commonly used incompatible response that is paired with physiological hyper arousal symptoms, such as high blood pressure (Blanchard et al., 1989). Relaxation techniques can be used to reduce anxiety experienced in a particular situation prior to the re-experiencing of that situation. This is done through a process called systematic desensitization. In this procedure, the client imagines the anxiety-producing situation, breaking it down into a series of steps, which progress from the least anxiety-producing to the most anxiety-producing (Wodarski & Bagarozzi, 1979). When relaxed, the client imagines the least anxiety-producing aspect of the situation. For instance, in the case of a client who is experiencing anxiety over returning to the hospital for additional chemotherapy treatments, a first step might be for the client to imagine getting in to the car to go to the hospital. If the client becomes anxious, he/she would proceed to the next step, such as driving up and seeing the hospital. The client would continue in this way, stopping to relax at each feeling of anxiety until the situation has been completed.

Operant Techniques

Operant behavior is viewed as voluntary behavior because it is not dependent upon environmental stimuli for its occurrence. Interpersonal behavior is usually considered to be an example of an operant behavior (Pinkerton et al., 1982). Operant conditioning attaches consequences to specific behaviors to affect the probability of whether or not the behaviors will be repeated in the future (Abramson, 1977). The operant model focuses on changing rates of behavior through the control of antecedents (discriminative stimuli) and/or consequences. Simply stated, positive reinforcers are used to increase behavior rates, and negative or neutral stimuli are used to reduce the behavior occurrence.

Positive reinforcement operates to increase behavior through the use of contingent rewards administered either by the client or by others. Praise and money are often used with powerful results. When contingency management is utilized, all aspects of the reward system should be clearly specified in a written contract, that is, what behaviors are to be reinforced, by whom, and how frequently (Pinkerton et al., 1982).

To reduce behavior, techniques such as punishment, extinction, and stimulus control are commonly used (Bandura, 1969). Punishment refers to the administration of an aversive stimulus after an undesirable response. Punishment should always be used in conjunction with positive reinforcement for desirable behavior (Pinkerton et al., 1982). For example, in weight control programs, aversive stimuli have been paired simultaneously with food stimuli. Aversive procedures are generally difficult for a client and the overall effectiveness is unclear (Wilson et al., 1987). For this reason, there is agreement among most social learning theorists that these procedures are best restricted to extreme situations.

Extinction is a procedure whereby the reinforcement that sustains a maladaptive behavior is withheld when the behavior is exhibited (Wodarski, 1985). For example, to decrease a client's "sick-role" behavior, attending staff members would ignore complaining and demands for special attention. For the procedure to be maximally effective, the staff would, at the same time, give the patient attention for "wellness" behavior.

Stimulus control is a procedure that is based on the consideration that most behavior occurs in specific situations rather than at all times and involves removing the discriminative stimuli (antecedent) that enhances the occurrence of that behavior. Removing favorite foods from the house or restricting the times and places where eating can occur are examples of stimulus control strategies for weight loss. Stimulus control can also focus on response prevention, as in the case of the bulimic who is instructed to eat large amounts of food without responding by vomiting (Agras et al., 1989).

Cognitive Techniques

One of the greatest problems with social learning theory is in the maintenance of the behavior change after the termination of treatment. Cognitive techniques can aid greatly in this maintenance since clients are able to practice behaviors in a variety of settings. Both overt and covert positive reinforcement are techniques that must comply with the same laws of utilization (Wodarski, 1985). Their difference is that in covert reinforcement, the behavior and its reinforcement are imagined by the client (Cautela, 1970a, 1970b, 1970c, 1970d).

The premise behind covert reinforcement is that when an imagined behavior is followed by an imagined pleasant stimulus, the likelihood of the behavior's occurrence increases. Another process, covert extinction, works in a similar way. In this process the probability of a behavior's reoccurrence is decreased by imagining that it is followed by a non-reinforcing event (Cautela, 1971). This process is often used in combination with covert positive reinforcement in order to replace non-adaptive behaviors with adaptive ones (Wodarski & Bagarozzi, 1979). The procedures for performing overt reinforcement are almost identical to those of covert reinforcement. In both techniques, homework becomes a very important component of the treatment, as the client must agree to practice the imaged scenes a specific number of times per day and keep a record of this. For example, clients can covertly positively reward themselves for medication compliance (Levy, 1987).

Changes in behavior which are brought about through social learning theory are of little use to the client if he/she is unable to maintain these changes after treatment is terminated. If cognitive behavioral techniques can be used to increase the maintenance and generalization of the behavior change, then they will have done much to increase the usefulness of social learning therapy. An added bonus of therapy is the increase in self-esteem which often accompanies successful attempts to modify one's own health behaviors through self-induced therapeutic techniques and increases the probability of maintenance of the health behavior.

Treatment Process

Although the above techniques are well researched and have been shown to increase wellness behaviors, more efforts need to be directed to address the deficiency in the area of developing individualized treatment plans with the client. Treatment plans tailored to the individual enable the addressing of individual needs and thus increase the probability of adherence. Social workers must be added to the list of professionals who formulate and administer these treatment plans in the primary care physician's office in order to adequately incorporate social learning techniques and preventative efforts (Berkman et al., 1988; Coulter & Hancock, 1989; Leukefield, 1989; Marshack et al., 1988).

Assessment is critical to the process of developing a treatment plan. The social worker who has been included as a member of the interdisciplinary team should assess the individual's behaviors that are placing him/her at risk for the development of specific health problems. They should then discuss methods for reducing and/or extinguishing those behaviors and the development and maintenance of healthy lifestyle behaviors. Methods should be carefully chosen which are acceptable to both the therapist and the client. At this point, the therapist's knowledge is very important. It is crucial to be able to predict, at least to a certain extent, whether or not the individual will be responsive to a particular treatment. The best approach is one that employs a multi-intervention that covers all possible variables (Shannon, 1989).

The therapist and the client will work together to formulate the treatment goals. That the client be allowed to have a great deal of input into these goals is of paramount importance in behavioral treatments, since participants are required to be more active in the change process than are participants in other treatment approaches (McClelland, 1989). Appropriate expectations for behavioral changes should be developed along with the confidence that the client can change. It is the client who will carry out such assignments as recording, counting, monitoring, and rehearsing. These assignments make the client continually aware of his/her behaviors. The role of the social worker is to ensure that the treatment goals are stated in terms of specific, observable behaviors that are to be increased, decreased, or acquired and that appropriate interventions are implemented. This aids both the therapist and the client in keeping their efforts focused and is also important for evaluation of outcomes (Hilarski & Wodarski, 2001).

Due to the specific nature of behavioral treatments, it is crucial to focus on the acquisition or change of one behavior before attempting other desired behavior change and to slowly build to the more difficult ones. This ordering is beneficial because the small successes increase the client's confidence in the ability to control his/her own behaviors.

Most of the efforts in health related behavioral treatments have been directed at decreasing the behaviors that constitute a health risk to the individual. While this is most necessary, treatment efforts should not stop there. Treatment is not complete until the extinguished or reduced behaviors have been replaced by an increase in or acquisition of wellness behaviors. The lifestyle changes that are established through the addition of one wellness behavior often lay the groundwork for others. In this way, one health promoting behavior change leads to the increase in or acquisition of other health promoting behaviors and to additional health benefits. This is one of the greatest benefits of the inclusion of the social worker to the primary care physician's treatment team, as the social worker is skilled in the interventions that lead to behavior change.

Analysis of Social Work Practice: Economic Perspective

Cost Analysis: Cost analysis has gained increasing support as an important aspect of program evaluation. In addition to being concerned with the extent to which social service programs define and meet measurable objectives, evaluators must also be concerned with the cost of such programs. Even before the series of economic recessions, there was increased pressure on social work administrators to be "accountable." Gross (1980) describes two elements of accountability as the need for social workers to "exhibit that what they do is effective, i.e. that social workers are able to achieve socially valued goals, and that these goals are realized efficiently, i.e. in the cheapest way possible" (p. 31).

With cutbacks in federal funds for social services and the shifts of responsibility for many programs to the states, agency administrators will increasingly be concerned with issues of cost in order to begin new programs, to maintain existing levels of funding, and in many cases, to retain any level of funding at all. Administrators need information related to program costs, as well as program outcomes in order to compete successfully for scarce resources. They also need such information in order to make hard decisions about internal programming, that is, what adopted from the fields of business and economics has been cited as useful in facilitating such decision making (Levin, 1983).

Cost Benefits: Cost-benefit analysis is a process through which program costs and effects (benefits) are identified and quantified. Both costs and benefits are expressed in dollar amounts and then compared. If benefits exceed costs, the program is considered worthy of funding, assuming no limitation of funds.

Where there is a limitation of funds, a cost-benefit analysis can indicate where the most impact can be gotten for the dollar. Thus, cost-benefit analysis can be used to establish funding priorities. According to Stokey and Zeckhauser, "the fundamental rule of cost-benefit criteria is to select the alternative that produces the greatest net benefit" (1978, p. 137). Thus, cost-benefit analysis is concerned with maximizing gain for marginal input.

Cost-Effectiveness: Cost-effectiveness analysis differs from cost-benefit analysis in that it requires that a monetary value be assigned to program costs, but not to program impacts or benefits. The assumption behind this approach is that program objectives are based on society's willingness or desire to achieve certain goals. Thus, decision making is focused, not on which objective to work toward, but on identifying which program alternative will help meet the already identified objective in the most effective way. Cost-effectiveness analysis cannot help establish program priorities but can help "find the most effective way of obtaining priorities by some other means" (Buxbaum, 1981). Benefits, while not measured in dollar terms, are specified in certain non-monetary units, such as number of foster care children returned to their biological families, or recidivism rates. Cost-effectiveness analysis allows one to determine how many units of benefits are associated with alternative program approaches to reaching the same objectives.

Discussion: Evaluation of service effectiveness has been an ongoing problem for social agencies. Criteria for assessment of service effectiveness are difficult to establish. Such criteria are often tied to theories of human behavior, which are either explicitly or implicitly used as rationale for various intervention approaches and programs (Wodarski, 2000). Many of these theories have yet to be systematically evaluated as to their relationship to practice effectiveness. Perhaps the one criterion which can be used universally is the extent to which utilization of a specific theory and its practice implications produces desired outcomes in client behaviors (Fischer, 1971, 1978; Wodarski & Feldman, 1973). However, even when such a criterion can be specified, problems of measurement arise.

Efforts have been made to develop measures to assess client outcome which may be related to service provision (i.e., Hudson, 1982; Rittner & Wodarski, 1995). While many practitioners are using these and similar measures on an individual basis with clients, few agencies have instituted such measures as a means of evaluating overall agency effectiveness. This area of agency effectiveness, as measured by outcomes of service provision, will require continuing attention and additional research in the future. Without such documentation, it will be difficult for administrators to justify high cost programs or services in times of resource scarcity in the managed care environments.

Increasing emphasis on agency evaluation will necessitate that schools of social work develop curricula which will address multiple aspects of agency assessment from a practical point of view. Evaluation skills must be taught which will enable future graduates to develop and implement various types of assessment. Continuing education and in-service training programs can be developed which will develop these competencies in persons already occupying agency positions.

The comprehensive agency evaluation must encompass many different perspectives and foci. It must also utilize data from various sources including consumers, workers, and community service providers, as well as information from the accounting department.

The agency which engages in the differing types of assessment can, over a period of time, develop a holistic view of overall agency functioning, which identifies both areas of weakness and strength.

Cost of Social Work Services: From a cost standpoint, the intervention that social service systems have chosen is extremely costly and highly unproductive for both client and practitioner (Thyer & Wodarski, 1998). The empirical literature indicates that services should be structured in a short-term manner (Dulmus & Wodarski, 1996). Taking the following as the unit of analysis, for MSW beginning social worker earning $33,000 direct salary and 0.32 fringe benefits equaling $8,000, 32 hours of intervention will cost:

Salary:	$33,000
Total possible workable days per year:	52 × 5 = 260
× 8 hrs/day	= 2080
25% subtracted for holidays, administrative tasks	= 2080
	0.75
	= 1560
Cost per billable hour:	1560
	$33,000 = $21.00/hr
32 hrs. × $21.00/hr	= $672.00

From the calculation, 32 hours of services would cost $672.00. Thus, the possible savings realized through prevention are obvious.

Nevertheless, issues of accountability, ethical pressures, and data on practice effectiveness provide the impetus for integration. It is time to stop questioning and criticizing and apply the existing research to develop a rational framework among our many interests within the varying levels of social work.

Cost-Specific Treatment Analysis

1. *Substance Abuse*: "A new longitudinal study that proves beyond a shadow of a doubt what you have known intuitively all along: Substance Abuse treatment is cost-effective. Now there is proof. Treatment completed in Oregon saved the state $83 million over a 3-year period. For every dollar spent on completed treatment, the state saved at least $56.00 in reduced costs of welfare, food stamps, Medicaid, crime and imprisonment. How is that for putting a dollar value on treatment!" (Pelosi, 1996, p. 1129).

2. *Mental Health*: Mental disorders have a devastating impact on a significant number of Americans of all ages and socioeconomic levels. Congress has received testimony that as many as one third of American adults will suffer from a diagnosable mental disorder at some point in their lives, and an estimated 20 percent of the population has a mental disorder at any given time. An estimated 12 percent of the nation's 63 million children and adolescents suffer from one or more mental disorders. Alzheimer's disease affects over 4 million older Americans, and at least 15 percent of the elderly in nursing homes are clinically depressed.

In addition to the cost of human suffering and lost opportunity, mental disorders place an extraordinary burden on the financial resources of the country. In 1990, the economic cost of mental disorders, excluding the cost of alcohol abuse, was estimated at $98 billion, and the economic cost of drug abuse was estimated at an additional $66 billion. Despite these enormous expenditures, it is estimated that only 10–30 percent of individuals in need receive appropriate treatment (Pelosi, 1996).

A noteworthy effort to gather cost-effective data has already been made by National Institute of Mental Health (NIMH)-funded investigators. For example, Amiram Vinokur, Ph.D., and colleagues at the University of Michigan Preventive Intervention Research Center showed that an experimentally tested program for the unemployed workers reduced symptoms of depression and helped them find better paying, more satisfying jobs. Per participant, the program cost about $286 while netting an additional $1,128 in Federal and State taxes paid (Muehrer, 1996).

Economic Rationale for the Behavioral Health Social Worker

Following are illustrations of the cost-benefit analysis that supports the use of behavioral health social workers. In the first study, Yale researchers report on the costs associated with the two treatment conditions.

Was There a Cost Advantage for the Day Hospital with Crisis/Respite Care Program?

The day hospital with crisis/respite care condition was 20 percent less expensive than traditional inpatient care (mean cost = $33,917 vs. $26,820). The major differences were in the lengths of stay and costs of the index admissions; day hospital patients averaged 18.8 days compared with 25.5 days for inpatients, with costs that were 43 percent less for the former.

Did the Cost Advantage Apply to All Patients?

The authors report that patients in each diagnostic group were treated less expensively in day hospital/crisis respite program than those with comparable diagnosis assigned to the inpatient hospital, although differences for psychotic patients were smaller than for those who had mood disorders and were dually diagnosed with substance abuse disorders.

Where Did the Cost Differences Lie?

Direct service staff costs were roughly equal for the two conditions, which suggest that equivalent treatment intensity accounted for equal effectiveness in outcomes. The authors found the biggest absolute and relative differences in resource expenditures relate to operating costs. Such expenses were twice as high for inpatient care, averaging $13,063 compared with $6,618 for day hospital/crisis respite care.

What Do the Authors Recommend?

They conclude that hospitalizing most voluntary patients with uncomplicated psychiatric distress cannot be defended on the grounds of either effectiveness

Table 1.1 Average Costs by Diagnosis

Diagnosis	Inpatient	Day Hospital/Crisis Respite
Psychosis	$29,342	$25,731
Affective Disorder	$28,508	$17,942
Dual Diagnosis	$27,756	$17,652

or cost. Instead they call for effective methods for matching patients' needs with service offerings.

As shown in their cost analysis, maintaining psychiatric hospitals is expensive, and not all patients need the full array of services offered there, although the authors do caution that alternatives to hospitalization do not entirely replace the need for psychiatric hospitals (Sledge et al., 1996).

Child Welfare

Tiffany Field, Ph.D., and colleagues at the University of Miami Medical School found that 15 minutes of tactile stimulation three times a day increased premature infants' weight gain, responsiveness to social stimulation, and development at eight months of age. In addition, infants receiving the stimulation went home sooner than controls, reducing hospitals' costs an average of $3,000 per infant.

David Olds, Ph.D., and colleagues at the University of Rochester found that, in contrast to comparison services, prenatal and infancy home visitation improved a wide range of maternal and child health outcomes among poor, unmarried, teenaged women bearing their first children in a semi-rural county in upstate New York. By the time the children were 4 years of age, the average per family government savings were $1,772 for the sample as a whole, and $43,498 for low-income families. These savings do not take into account the additional health and social benefits of the program to participants (Muehrer, 1996).

Pre-School

A well-documented study traced the long-term consequences of an extensive program that offered child care and family support to low-income families in Syracuse, New York, during the first five years of their children's lives (Lally et al., 1988). A follow-up study ten years later compared children who had participated in the program with children from similar backgrounds who had not (Lally et al., 1988). The girls who had participated in the study were doing far better. In school, the boys who had participated were committing fewer and less severe criminal offenses, and all participants were more likely to remain in school than were their peers who had not participated in the study.

An additional study, conducted in Connecticut, followed two groups of low-income families with infants and toddlers (Provence & Naylor, 1983). One group received a coordinated set of health and social services; the other did not. At the ten-year follow-up, children in the first group were less likely to require special education, were likely to have better school attendance, and were better liked by their teachers than were children in the second group. In addition, more of the mothers in the first group had achieved self-sufficiency, completed more schooling, and had given birth to fewer subsequent children than the mothers in the second group. Per family, families in the second group received, on average, almost $3,000 more per year in welfare and special education services than did the first group.

In the 1990s the Carnegie Corporation and ZERO TO THREE/National Center for Clinical Infant Programs, began campaigns to inform the U.S. public about what helps and what hinders early development by publicizing the results of studies such as those described above. Such campaigns are costly, but unless policy makers and the public are made to understand, in clear and concise terms, the benefits of specific services, important programs will not receive the attention, support, and funding they require.

Behavioral Health Social Work: A Means to a Solution

The previous discussions suggest a new focus on solving health problems, a focus that centers on prevention through theory, assessment, intervention, and outcomes. The authors propose that behavioral health social work also offers a means for training practitioners to be able to solve health problems.

Behavioral health social work involves the systematic application of interventions derived from learning theory supported by empirical evidence to achieve behavior changes in clients resulting in better health. The behavioral health social worker must possess both theoretical knowledge and an empirical perspective regarding the nature of human behavior and the principles that influence behavioral change. The worker must be capable of translating this knowledge into concrete behavioral operations for practical use in a variety of practice settings. Therefore, in order to be an effective practitioner, the behavioral health social worker must possess a solid behavioral science knowledge base, as well as a variety of behavioral skills. Moreover, a thorough grounding in research methodology will enable the behavioral health social worker to evaluate the therapeutic interventions, a necessary requisite of managed care practice. Since the rigorous training of the behavioral health social worker equips her/him to assess and evaluate any intervention procedure that she/he has instituted, there is continual evaluation that provides corrective feedback to the practitioner. For the behavioral health social worker, theory, practice, and evaluation are all part of one intervention process. The arbitrary division of theory, intervention, and research, which does not facilitate therapeutic effectiveness and improved clinical procedures, is eliminated.

Implications for Social Work Practice

Managed care does and will have a profound impact on the way that services are delivered, and on the duration of those services. While social workers may view these time limitations as a decrease in their role and ability to be effective, they should instead welcome the opportunity to become educated about empirically validated brief intervention methods, and to utilize their assessment skills. The implementation of managed care has hindered social work provision of long-term service, but has enhanced social work effectiveness in screening and assessing client needs (Thyer & Wodarski, 1998).

Social workers can deal with the psychosocial and environmental aspects of illness. The link between mental health and somatic illness has become clear. Social workers have knowledge and training in the recognition and treatment of mental health problems that both medical specialists and physicians lack (Thyer & Wodarski, 1998).

Social Work Role

- Assess patient/client and family for ability to follow through on treatment plan.
- Support client through assessment, diagnosis, treatment, rehabilitation, etc.
- Guide clients through the system (what is covered, what is not, and to what extent).
- Educate and inform client and family members about the specific illness, coping techniques, outlook, etc.
- Address behavioral, emotional, or mental problems that may hinder decision making around the illness.
- Identify, discuss, and obtain entitlement benefits.
- Identify and facilitate linkages to appropriate non-medical resources (support groups, emergency food/housing, family/marital/couple/individual counseling, etc.).
- Share knowledge about the client and the family system with the team to ensure their ability to effectively care for the client.
- Advocate for patients who are dissatisfied with their care.

(Adapted from Berkman, 1996)

Profiling the Behavioral Health Social Worker

Behavioral social workers possess both theoretical knowledge and conceptual understanding about the nature of human behaviors in the principles of behavior change. They must also be capable of translating this knowledge and understanding into concrete behavioral operations for practical use in a variety of health care settings. In order to be an effective practitioner, therefore, the behavioral health social worker must possess a solid knowledge base as well as have a variety of behavioral skills.

> The present study surveyed graduate program training directors in clinical psychology, counseling psychology, and social work about the training opportunities available for their graduate students. Almost 60% of the respondents indicated that they provide some type of training related to managed care.
>
> (Daniels et al., 2002: 587)

This study shows that graduate programs are still behind where they should be in implementing programs that will allow students to participate in managed care settings.

Knowledge Base

The body of knowledge that the behavioral social worker must possess in order to an effective practitioner should include the following:

- A thorough understanding of the scientifically derived principles and theories of human learning as they relate to human behavior, personality formation, the development and maintenance of interpersonal relationship, and behavior change.
- An ability to conceptualize a client's behavior and to make accurate behavioral assessment based upon the principles and theories and to make accurate behavioral assessment based upon the principles and theories so that the appropriate techniques can be developed and effective programs formulated to bring about the desired behavioral acquisitions, modifications, or extinctions of unwanted behaviors for those clients who request such changes.
- An ability to understand how these principles of learning and behavior changes can be applied on a broad scale to alleviate the social and societal problems.
- An understanding of how this knowledge of human behavior and these principles of learning can be utilized in a variety of contexts and settings, for example, with individuals, in groups, among family members, and within large organizations and institutions as well as in naturalistic settings.
- The ability to evaluate objectively any treatment procedure and outcome and to formulate new treatment strategies when those formulated originally had been proven ineffective.

Key Impact Areas for a Behavioral Health Model

The main influence pushing primary care behavioral integration is the need to control medical costs that directly arise from psychosocial or mental health factors by providing quality treatment. This means that the activities of the behavioral health clinician need to be focused on achieving four main outcomes:

1 Enhancing the short-term critical outcomes of primary care, health, and mental health interventions for patients with mental health or emotional concerns.
2 Enhancing longer-term outcomes in patients who have recurrent, chronic, or progressive medical or mental health conditions.

3   Controlling medical utilization and costs by providing appropriate behavioral health support to patients who need ongoing social support or who have chronic and treatment resistant mental and medical problems (Cummings et al., 1996).
4   Provide accurate assessment of the psychosocial aspects of ailments and integration of services.

Emerging Roles for Behavioral Interventions in Primary Care

According to Thyer and Wodarski (1998), there is every reason to believe that behaviorally based interventions can dramatically increase the quality of mental health care provided in the general medical setting (cf. Strosahl, 1995). First, the behavior therapy model is rich in diagnostically driven treatment approaches. Many behavioral interventions were developed to treat specific mental disorders, and only later evolved into generalized behavior change

Table 1.2 Core Clinical Services in Primary Health Care

Service	Primary
1. Behavior health consultation	First visit by a patient for a general evaluation; focus diagnostic and functional evaluation, recommendation for treatment and forming limited behavior change goals; involves assessing patients at risk because of some likely stress event.
2. Behavior health follow-up	Secondary visits by a patient to support a behavior change plan or treatment started by a provider* on the basis of earlier consultation; often in tandem with planned provider visits.
3. Triage/Liaison	Visit designed to determine appropriate mental health specialty referral outside of primary care setting; usually a single visit.
4. Compliance enhancement	Visit designed to help patients comply with medication initiated provider; focus on education, addressing negative beliefs, or strategies for coping with side effects.
5. Relapse prevention	Visit designed to maintain stable functioning in a patient who has responded to previous treatment; often spaced at long intervals.
6. Speciality consultation	Visit part of a condensed speciality patient education package conducted by the consultant; visit usually linked to planned provider visits; involves 4 to 6 short sessions; usually reserved for mental conditions such as panic disorder or major depression.
7. Community resource	Visit designed to educate patient about available community resources in a particular area (i.e. support groups for caregivers).

strategies. For example, relaxation training was originally a key strategy in systematic desensitization, but is now employed in a myriad of behaviorally based intervention packages both in and out of medical settings.

Second, behavioral interventions have demonstrated clinical effectiveness with a wide range of mental disorders and psychosocial problems commonly encountered in primary care. Major depression, panic disorder, generalized anxiety disorder, chronic pain, and somatization disorder are common conditions seen in medical practice, and can be addressed with empirically supported, time-effective behavior therapies (Thyer & Wodarski, 1998).

Third, the behavioral approach is equally facile at addressing health and illness behaviors (cf. Friedman et al., 1995; Strosahl, 1994). Behavioral interventions are arguably the most effective strategies for promoting health (i.e., myocardial infarction).

Fourth, the behavioral approach can be expanded to fit family or relationship realities just as easily as it can be applied to the individual patient.

Table 1.2 (continued)

Service	Primary
8. Case management	Visit designed to support functioning in a chronically distressed patient; visit intervals long but continuing; often part of a visit package that is designed to reduce unplanned medical visits.
9. Behavioral medicine	Visit designed to assess patient in managing a chronic medical condition or to tolerate invasive or uncomfortable medical procedure; focus may be on lifestyle issues or health risk factors among patients at risk (i.e. smoking cessation, weight loss).
10. Conjoint consultation	Visit with provider and patient designed to address an issue of concern to both; often involves addressing an issue between them.
11. Provider consultation	Face to face with physician to discuss patient care issues; often involves "curbside" consultation; can include formal case conference with provider and health care team.
12. Team building	Conference with one or more members of health care team to address peer relationships, job stress issues, or process of care concerns.
13. On demand consultation	Phone or face to face contact with provider, usually "emergent"; focus on addressing an immediate care issue.

* Provider means any primary care giver such as a physician, physician's assistant, clinical nurse specialist, registered nurse, licensed practical nurse, women's health care specialist.

Pertinent family or relationship reinforcements can be addressed directly within a learning framework. This is important because primary care medicine is not only oriented toward the individual patient, but also emphasizes health and well-being in family living.

Fifth, behavioral technology is easily transferable to the patient, using patient education and self-care models that are already widely employed in the primary care management of chronic diseases, such as diabetes. These models focus on teaching each patient self-management and behavior change skills, while placing more responsibility on the patient for executing these behaviors.

Finally, primary care providers tend to be very pragmatic in their patient interventions, and naturally gravitate to using behavioral techniques (cf. Robinson, 1995; Robinson et al., 1995). Therefore, the overlap between natural physician practice and behavioral strategies makes behavioral interventions very acceptable in the primary care setting (see Table 1.2 for elucidation of roles).

Summary

The health care industry is changing rapidly, and with it will come changes to managed health care as we know it. This addresses a fundamental paradigm shift with far reaching implications for the effectiveness of health care, the cost-efficiency of health care systems, and the service integration of systems (Masia et al., 1997). These changes are affecting previously segregated delivery systems, specifically those of health and mental health. Increased costs and proposed budget cuts are forcing segregated systems into an overall integrated delivery system with the intent of providing more adequate care (Wodarski, 2000).

It has been increasingly shown that health care costs and the effective management of health care are of primary importance and concern to federal, state, and local governments. It is necessary to develop innovative, successful, and cost-effective assessments and treatment procedures. This text proposed such procedures by defining the problems to be addressed, applying research and studies for support, and presenting an innovative model for cost-effective and integrated managed health care combined with empirically based psychosocial intervention and prevention.

Finally, a profile of the Behavioral Health Social Worker was defined describing the abilities of an effective behavioral social worker. Among the required attributes are (1) the depth of an acceptable knowledge base, (2) the behavioral skills necessary for an intellectual and conceptual understanding of theories of human development and learning, and (3) the utilization of techniques necessary to bring about behavioral changes in clinical practice. From these key characteristics, a foundation is established for the emerging roles of behavioral interventions in primary care. These interventions will ultimately increase the quality of psychosocial health care in terms of access and integration while effectively controlling medical costs.

2 The Integrated Service Delivery System*

Introduction

In addition to regular routine health care, many patients who present in primary physician offices suffer from psychological and psychosocial problems, which may be impacting their physical health. "The Integrated Service Delivery System," incorporates state-of-the-art rapid assessment techniques and computer technology, appropriate interventions matched to assessed patient deficits, and coordination and follow-up in providing an innovative and progressive approach to assist the physician in management of patients' alcohol and substance abuse, mental health and psychological stresses affecting their health. This comprehensive approach to patient management incorporates a bachelors' level social worker (BSW), with appropriate Master of Science in Social Work (MSSW) supervision, within the physician's office to provide assessment, crisis management, time limited psychological interventions, and linkage to social agencies and other professionals in the community to address issues related to psychosocial problems impacting physical health. The model is cost-effective and ultimately better meets the patient's health care needs.

Problems and stresses including: domestic violence, parenting issues, poverty, drug/alcohol abuse, and individual mental health issues can instigate new health concerns or exacerbate already existing health problems. Often, these problems go unrecognized in a health care system that views such problems as falling outside the physician's scope of practice as well as not being adequately prepared to detect them. Ultimately, if not addressed in timely manner, these problems over time can impact a patient's physical health and can result in higher health care costs. Many patients, whose only health care contact is provided through their primary physician, never receive the psychosocial treatment necessary for overall health care and well-being. A simple referral by their physician to social service agencies and/or social work professionals could ensure this.

* Chapter written with assistance of: Teressa Gregory.

Intervention for psychosocial problems that have the potential to impact a person's physical health is necessary, and in the long run cost-effective. The provider constituency in primary care includes a rather bewildering number of physicians (e.g., family practice, general internal medicine, obstetrics-gynecology, pediatrics) and allied health care groups (physician's assistant, clinical nurse specialists, registered and licensed nurses, women's health care specialist), all of whom provide routine medical care and encounter patients with mental disorders or significant psychosocial stresses. Indeed, research indicates that half of all the formal mental health care in the United States is delivered solely by these providers (Rieger et al., 1993). This would indicate that individual treatment is primarily limited to pharmacological intervention. This is unfortunate when one considers that empirically proven cognitive and behavioral interventions are now available to treat an array of mental diagnosis, in combination or in lieu of medication.

Eighty percent of the population visit their primary care physician at least annually. However, only about half of individuals with diagnosable mental disorders seek mental health care from any professional. Those patients with psychological or psychosocial concerns seek instead medical care generated by physical symptoms of distress (Smith et al., 1995). Kroenke and Mangelsdorf (1989) found that of the ten most common physical complaints in primary care, 85 percent end up with a known diagnosable organic etiology during a three-year follow-up period (Kroenke & Mangelsdorf, 1989).

The Bachelor-Level Social Worker and the Integrated Service Delivery Model

The health care industry is changing rapidly and with it will come changes to managed care as it is now known. These changes are affecting previously segregated delivery systems, specifically those of health and mental health. Increased costs and proposed budget cuts are forcing segregated systems into an overall integrated delivery system. "The Integrated Service Delivery System" employs a model that changes the policies and procedures that are presently employed in most primary physician's practices. The model incorporates a bachelor's level social worker (BSW) with MSSW supervision into the physician's office.

The BSW professional offers a unique contribution to medical practice. To attain a Master of Social Work (MSW) an individual must complete two years of graduate education (60 hours beyond the bachelor's degree). The curriculum incorporates courses that examine the person in the environment, generally utilizing a bio-psychosocial approach, with many schools of social work offering a concentration specific to health care. Additionally, most states license social workers. With malpractice being a concern to all professionals, malpractice insurance is readily available for social workers to purchase through the National Association of Social Workers.

"The Integrated Service Delivery System" (Appendix A) utilizes a BSW who administers state-of-the-art rapid assessment to patients referred by the physician, to identify psychological stressors that may be impacting the patient's health.

In addition to assessment, the BSW would provide linkage to social agencies and other professionals to address specific areas of concern identified in the assessment. Referral agencies would provide progress reports to the MSW to allow follow-up and coordination of services. The MSW would also be available to provide crisis management, time limited psychological interventions and indicated, and promoted, prevention agenda (Dulmus & Wodarski, 1997).

The challenges facing health care today demand accurate mental health assessment and diagnosis as well as testing bio-psychosocial interventions (Keigher, 1997) which the MSW is qualified to perform. Interventions provided by the MSW are often reimbursable by the patient's insurance, which could ultimately not only cover the additional expense of employing an MSW, but also result in a profit margin for the physician, while more importantly better meeting the needs of the patients. An MSW in the physician's office would certainly be a strong addition to the medical team.

Rapid Assessment

The model incorporates rapid assessment techniques, which have become increasingly popular with practitioners and agencies. The trend to use rapid assessment techniques has been in response to recent requests by funding agencies to produce evidence that clients are reaching their stated goals and for proof that programs are effective in treating clients. Practitioners and agencies have come to realize that the use of rapid assessment instruments is instrumental in meeting these two important aspects of managed care. In the managed care arena, no doubt rapid assessment techniques have been associated with the recent requests by funding agencies to have evidence that clients are reaching their stated goals and that programs are effective in treating their clients. In the managed care arena, no doubt rapid assessment technology would be a welcomed tool.

Social workers have begun to realize the ability of rapid assessment instruments to collect larger quantities as well as providing better quality data. Studies have consistently found that these instruments are easily administered, cost-effective and can provide reliable client data (McMahon, 1984: Rittner & Wodarski, 1995; Streever et al., 1984). In addition rapid assessment instruments are more objective than personal interviews, in that the personal biases of the worker are reduced and the subjective nature of assessment as a whole is decreased. Flowers et al. (1993) found that the clients who utilized rapid assessment instruments throughout treatment, made more improvement on their goals, terminated from treatment less often and were in general, more satisfied with treatment. These instruments have also been noted to obtain more information from clients in a shorter amount of time. Consequently, rapid assessment is more efficient as well as more accurate.

Social workers, who work with children, adults, and families with multiple problems, need to assess multiple sources of data across and beyond family systems. At the present time, many professionals use clinical interviews, personal judgment, and assumptions to make decisions about services and treatment needs. There are multiple problems associated with conducting assessment in this manner which the Integrated Service Delivery System would address. The use of the Integrated Service Delivery System would reduce this potential of subjectivity and provide the physician with a package of easy to use assessment instruments, which then could be administered by the BSW. By utilizing these techniques, the BSW can readily assess problems that may impact the individual patient's overall physical health. The patient would be assessed for alcohol and drug problems, mental illness, family violence, child abuse, housing needs, nutrition, financial problems, etc. This information would then be utilized to provide the patient with an individualized treatment plan and appropriate referrals. By utilizing these valid assessment instruments, the social worker increases his/her chance of making an accurate evaluation of the client's psychosocial needs that may be impacting physical health. In using this holistic approach all aspects of the patient's emotional, mental, and physical health would be addressed resulting in a more efficient and effective assessment.

Additionally, information gathered through the use of rapid assessment instruments has the potential to be a multi-agency document which further reduces the cost of each client consent; the assessment could be forwarded to the service agencies where the client would be referred for additional or further treatment. This process would assist the service agencies by providing reliable information about the client's problems prior to the first meeting; it would also reduce replicated information gathering by the service agencies.

Computer Assistance

Computer technology is integral to the model; rapid assessment instruments can be completed by clients directly on the computer. The computer can then score these and generate a profile of potential areas of bio-psychosocial difficulties, which then can be stored on the computer and (with consent) forwarded to all referred service providers. This procedure has been proven to be an accurate way to obtain information and is quicker and easier for clients and workers to use (Flowers, et al., 1993; Hays et al., 1993).

Computers could be utilized at every level of the health care system to improve speed as well as accuracy. At the level of intake, the bachelor level social worker can begin to generate a physical psychosocial file that could be directly stored on the computer. Included in this file would be rapid assessment results, treatment plans and client goals, referrals to service providers, client progress reports and client terminations. The computer system can assist in client monitoring and improve the overall integration of services. The following provides a more detailed description of how a computer system will further integration and efficiency.

Patient files would be stored directly on computer and would include the rapid assessment results, treatment plans, patient goals, service provider referrals, progress reports and patient termination. The computer system could assist in patient monitoring and improvement of overall service integration. In addition, this system would incorporate the patient's complete medical file for easier access for review and update.

Additionally, this information could be readily accessed and used to develop termination plans. Upon termination, the computer generates an overall outcome evaluation. It reports statistically what improvements occurred in what areas. This allows the social worker a more objective means to validate termination. The outcome evaluation also identifies difficulties within the system and provides an assessment of the entire delivery system. This information could also be used at a later date to assist the physician with improving professional skills, quality improvement, personal training, and integration. The computer can also help generate useful statistics, which could further assist with managed care reporting requirements.

The model client who is reported to the BSW and is subsequently designated a founded case, would be assigned a case manager. Due to the intensive case management of each case in this model, it would be essential for workers to have a limited number of clients in their caseload to ensure adequate time to provide necessary case coordination. Once a case has been founded, the case manager would be responsible to complete the intake and the initial assessment, utilizing the Service Provider Measurement Package (Appendix B) to determine the client's family's strengths and deficits. This measurement package includes the Hudson MPSI (Multi-Problem Screening Inventory) and family risk scale, FASI (Family Assessment Service Integrity), and if adolescents are involved, the MAAS (Multidimensional Adolescent Assessment Scale) as well.

In addition, an assessment of current services to which the client/family is linked would be able to be accessed (Appendix B). This information would be the basis of the Integrated Individual Service Plan (Appendix C). Development of this plan would begin with the BSW worker who would complete a problem identification assessment, problem selection, and goal development with the client.

Based on the identified deficits in the initial assessment, the case manager would acquire necessary releases and make referrals, on the client's behalf, to various service providers (i.e., substance abuse mental health, support collection, WIC (Women, Infants and Childrens Programs), legal aid, etc.) for further specific assessment and intervention. The service provider would provide diagnosis definition, objective creation and intervention delivery. They would utilize a standardized rapid assessment package to provide further assessment (Appendix B). Based on that assessment they would provide intervention/services as indicated (Appendix C) and record that information on a service technology form (Appendix D). In addition, they would complete and provide monthly Progress/Review Reports (Appendix E) to the MSW as to the client's progress. These reports would incorporate the intervention modality and technology utilized, along with the client's overall progress toward treatment goals. This report would allow the case manager to monitor the client's compliance and progress.

Each time a new issue was identified which required a referral, the service provider would refer the client back to the case manager who would then initiate the referral (Appendix A). This information flow would require strict adherence to ensure that service providers did not make referrals between themselves on the client's behalf as this would undermine the case manager's role and inhibit the model design.

The Physician's Integrated Service Delivery System proposes the use of rapid assessment instruments to provide intake and service agency workers with quick, accurate information on their clients. These instruments can provide quantifiable means of assessment that can significantly augment data collected through traditional procedures (Rittner & Wodarski, 1995). These instruments are essential for accurate assessment and hence effective intervention. In addition, these instruments are valuable planning, monitoring client change and outcome evaluation.

Appendix A: The Physician's Integrated Service Delivery System Referral Flow Chart

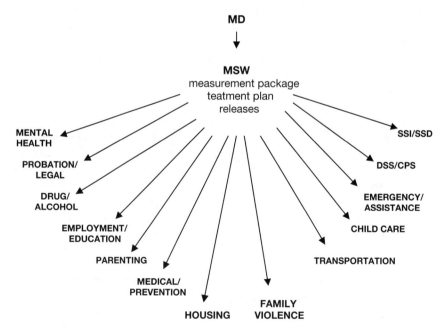

Appendix B: Service Providers Measurement Packages

CPS
MPSI

Childhood level of living scale

Mental Health/Crisis Services
MPSI
Symptom Checklist-SC
Reasons for Living Inventory

Drug & Alcohol
Miller SASSI
Hudson Index of Drug Involvement Scale

Medical/Dental/Prevention
Physical examination

Immediate Emergency Assistance
Yes/No qualifier

Housing
FASI housing subscale

Family Violence
MPSI
Partner Abuse Scale Physical (PASPH)
Partner Abuse Scale: Non-physical (PASNP)
Hwaiek-Sengstock Elder Abuse Screening Test

Parenting
The Knowledge of Behavior Principles as Applied to Children-
    (KBPAC)—Index of Parental Attitudes

Probation/Legal Support Collection
Yes/No qualifier

Employment/Education
TABE
CASAS
RAT

Transportation
Yes/No Qualifier

Child Care
Yes/No Qualifier

SSI/SSD
Yes/No Qualifier

DSS
FASI
Family Risk Scale

Appendix C: Integrated Individual Service Plan

Place a check next to the services which the client is already receiving and for those which the client needs a referral.

Services Already Received   **Services Needed**

Services Already Received	Services Needed	
_____	_____	(1) Mental Health Services
_____	_____	(2) Substance Abuse Services
_____	_____	(3) Probation/Legal Involvement
_____	_____	(4) Public Assistance Services
_____	_____	(5) Employment/Education Services
_____	_____	(6) Parenting Services
_____	_____	(7) Family Violence Services
_____	_____	(8) Medical/Prevention Services
_____	_____	(9) Housing Services
_____	_____	(10) Transportation Services
_____	_____	(11) Child Care Services
_____	_____	(12) Intensive/Crisis Services
_____	_____	(13) Child Protective Services

Appendix D: Service Technology Form

Mental Health

Modality:
_____ Individual Therapy
_____ Couple Therapy
_____ Family Therapy
_____ Group Therapy

Technology:
_____ Relaxation Training
_____ Assertiveness Training
_____ Anger Management
_____ Stress Management
_____ Problem-solving Skills
_____ Self-esteem Building Skills
_____ Supportive Therapy

Drug and Alcohol Services

Modality:
_____ Individual Therapy
_____ Couple Therapy

_____ Family Therapy
_____ Group Therapy

Technology:
_____ Relaxation Training
_____ Assertiveness Training
_____ Stress Management
_____ Problem-solving Skills
_____ Self-esteem Building Skills

Probation/Legal/Support Collection
Modality:
_____ Completed PINS petition
_____ Paternity – Filed Support order
_____ Filed for enforcement
_____ Legal Aid Assistance

Employment/Education
Modality:
_____ Individual Therapy
_____ Group Therapy

Technology:
_____ Assessment (including basic skills assessment)
_____ Job Seeking Skills
_____ Job Leads

Parenting
Modality:
_____ Individual Therapy
_____ Couple Therapy
_____ Family Therapy
_____ Group Therapy

Technology:
_____ Relaxation Training
_____ Stress Management
_____ Problem-solving Skills
_____ Supportive Therapy
_____ Behavior Modification Principles
_____ Child Development Education

Family Violence
Modality:
_____ Individual Therapy
_____ Couple Therapy

____   Family Therapy
____   Group Therapy

Technology:
____   Relaxation Training
____   Assertiveness Training
____   Anger Management
____   Stress Management
____   Problem-solving Skills

Medical/Prevention Services

Physical Examination completed:
____   Yes
____   No
____   Additional referrals needed

Housing

Modality:
____   Individual
____   Family

Technology:
____   Emergency Shelter
____   Permanent Housing
____   Security Deposit
____   1st Month Rent

Transportation

Provided:
____   Yes
____   No

Child Care

Provided:
____   Yes
____   No

Intensive/Crisis Services

Modality:
____   Individual Therapy
____   Couple Therapy
____   Family Therapy
____   Group Therapy

Technology:
____   Relaxation Training
____   Stress Management

____	Problem-solving Skills
____	Supportive Therapy
____	Assessment Diagnosis
____	Safety Planning

Appendix E: Progressive Review Report

Client Name: _____

ID: _____

DATE: _____

Linkage to referral was made?   (1) YES   (2) NO

Is client regularly attending program/appointments?   (1) YES   (1) NO

The client's outcome goal is?   (1) Progressing   (2) Unchanged

(3) Failing   (4) Completed

The client requires additional services?   (1) YES   (2) NO

If yes, check needed services:

____	Mental Health Services
____	Probation/Legal Support Collection
____	Drug & Alcohol Services
____	Employment/Education Services
____	Parenting Training
____	Medical/Dental/Prevention Services
____	Family Violence Services
____	Transportation Services
____	Intensive Management/Crisis Services
____	Child Care Services
____	Housing Services
____	SSI/SSD

3 Managed Care, Assessment Instruments, and Helping Professionals*

The stringent standards required by Managed Health Care have changed the way that service is delivered by all human service agencies. The managed care system now requires helping professionals (physicians, psychologists, social workers, etc.) to be accountable for the types of service they provide, the type of clientele that they serve, and the expense, duration, and outcome of the services provided. Part of being an accountable practitioner is working from an empirical basis in relation to interventions, data collection, and treatment process (Wodarski, 1997). This emphasis on accountability comes in response to the decreasing federal and state monetary and philosophical support (Wodarski, 1997). Therefore, professionals are required to work accurately, swiftly, empirically, and in a limited amount of time, while delivering services that are ever more effective and more cost efficient. The standardized require-ments of managed care have turned the profession toward creating rapid assessment instruments (RAIs) that are easy to administer, score, and complete without losing validity or reliability.

Many instruments exist that are reliable and valid when measuring one aspect of a problem or a particular diagnosis, however, the need is growing for an instrument that can provide the worker with a differential diagnosis for problems related to substance abuse or physical or mental health concerns. These will assist the professional in creating a quicker, more accurate assess-ment of problems, so that they can refer clients to the appropriate helping agent. RAIs would also highlight what areas might have compounded or contributing factors. The factors often remain unnoticed when helping professionals zero in on their own area of expertise; they may fail to notice problems in other areas. This approach requires a more collaborative and interactive component on the part of helping professionals. There is reason to believe that the interdisciplinary team approach can be an effective way to navigate through managed care systems (Resnick & Tighe, 1997). This type

* Chapter written with assistance of: Suzanne Vayda.

of assessment tool would also result in more appropriate and accurate referrals to different helping agents.

The changes that are occurring in the way social workers deliver services are largely attributable to the growth of managed care companies (Munson, 1996). In 2000, managed care companies covered 75 percent of insured people in the United States (Kiesler, 2000) as compared to 51 percent in 1995 and only 29 percent in 1990 (Munson, 1996). The changes that are being implemented through managed care companies come in response to the rising cost of health care in the United States (Berkman, 1996). In 1995, the cost constituted 15 percent of the gross national product for one year, which is equivalent to one trillion dollars (Shortell et al., 1995).

The goal of managed care is to alter the treatment process in hopes of reducing the amount of unnecessary health service utilization (Berkman, 1996). The treatment process currently experiences budget and utilization constraints. There are financial rewards for service providers who limit services, and pre-established treatment plan/goals with regular reviews are becoming the norm. The more powerful role of managed care organizations has also impacted the decision-making process regarding which services will be provided. In the past, exclusively physicians and clients made these decisions.

Interdisciplinary Team Model

The idea of using an interdisciplinary team approach to provide appropriate client care has become widespread (DeAngelis, 2005; Resnick & Tighe, 1997). The interdisciplinary team generally contains social workers, physicians, physician assistants, psychiatrists, and other paraprofessionals. Utilizing this model leads to more accurate diagnoses, more efficient use of professionals' time, a decrease in cost, and more appropriate client care (Resnick & Tighe, 1997). The interdisciplinary team approach requires the members of the team to work within their area of expertise, maximizing the use of their education. The enhanced function of the role differentiation in this model enables professionals to meet the needs of a greater number of clients at a lower cost (Resnick & Tighe, 1997). The cost reductions involved in the utilization of this model allow managed care companies to expand their scope in a greater attempt to achieve nationwide health care.

> Unless the complex social and medical needs of patients are recognized and unless a comprehensive package of services is provided based on an interdisciplinary health care model (including social workers), a majority of Americans will be underinsured or forced to pay significant additional fees for uncovered services or supplemental insurance
> (Mizrahi, 1993, p. 89)

The addition of social services and mental health services to the primary care practitioner will be beneficial to the patient in a variety of ways as well.

A common patient data system can be used enabling a better understanding of the person. An interdisciplinary team can also keep track of medications being taken, medical compliance and possible drug interactions (Kiesler, 2000).

RAIs Model for Differential Diagnosis

Short screening questionnaires have been found to have a reasonable degree of specificity and acceptable false-positive rates (Berwick et al., 1991). These measures have been found to be incorporated into the primary care setting and other agency intakes with ease. The hope is that they will achieve greater utilization in a more diverse range of practice settings than have longer versions of these questionnaires (Lairson et al., 1992). The increased usage of these instruments will result in an increased detection of alcohol related and mental health problems. This will pave the way for earlier intervention and more appropriate treatment (Berwick et al., 1991).

The top RAIs found effective in assessing difficulties in the fields of alcohol abuse, mental health, and physical health, are CAGE, the GHQ-12 or GSI-25, and DAPA. All of these scales can be implemented into a primary care setting and can yield rapid and accurate assessments, which allow for appropriate referrals to a worker on the team in a corresponding discipline. In addition, these instruments can be administered with ease, are simply scored, and are supported by empirical evidence of their validity and reliability.

Numerous findings reveal that primary care physicians often overlook significant mental disorders (Berwick et al., 1991) and alcohol abuse (Liskow & Campbell, 1995) in their patients (Lairson et al., 1992). Liskow and Campbell (1995) have found that an average of 20–30 percent of clients in clinical settings have alcohol-related problems and that physicians only detect between 10 and 50 percent of those afflicted. Of the patients with mental disorders, half or more go undiagnosed and untreated (Berwick et al., 1991). As a result, many of the presenting problems that patients are being treated for may be compounded by mental health and alcohol complications. Researchers have found a relationship between disability payments, schizophrenia, and substance abuse. Studies have also shown that substance abuse disorders affect individuals with disabilities other than mental illness (Bachman et al., 2004). Assessing for substance abuse issues is beneficial when there is mental illness or physical illness present.

CAGE

This RAI is comprised of four questions that relate directly to the effects of the individual's alcohol use. The questions require a "yes" or a "no" answer. The CAGE acronym represents the four areas highlighted in the instrument's questions. The questions are as follows: (1) Have you ever felt the need to *Cut* down on your drinking? (2) Are you ever *Annoyed* by others' criticisms of your drinking? (3) Have you ever felt *Guilty* about your drinking? (4) Have you ever needed a drink first thing in the morning to settle your nerves or relieve a hangover (*Eye opener*)? (Ewing & Rouse, 1970). This scale could improve its versatility by expanding its scope to include drug use as well. If this was done, the scale might read like this: (1) Have you ever felt the need to cut down on your drinking or drug use? (2) Are you ever annoyed by others' criticisms of your drinking or drug use? (3) Have you ever felt guilty about your drinking or drug use? (4) Have you ever needed to drink or use drugs (get high) first thing in the morning to settle your nerves or get you going? This minor adaptation of the scale greatly improves the scale's ability to be utilized with a wider array of clientele. Utilizing a scale like this would also eliminate some of the overlap that is found in the medical and psychiatric assessments, because it is shorter as well as reliable. Before an adaptation, the validity and reliability of this new measure must be ascertained to ensure that it will still be an accurate and reliable measure.

The cutting score for the CAGE scale is two or more affinitive responses, which indicates that alcohol abuse is an area of concern for the respondents. The CAGE scale has been found to be both valid and reliable in primary care as well as in general population surveys (Liskow & Campbell, 1995; Watson et al., 1995). An obvious strength of this measure is its length, which enables the professional to administer and score the responses accurately and in a short period of time. Due to the length of the CAGE scale, it is unable to provide much detail about the nature of the alcohol problem. Consequentially, for more specific assessment, CAGE should be employed along with another measure of a thorough interview. For purposes of detection, however, CAGE has been found very useful (Berwick et al., 1991; Watson et al., 1995). The scale has been found to have the highest rate of detecting alcohol dependence in 1994 (Watson et al., 1995). Although the model has been found to lack specificity regarding the stage of alcohol abuse, it was found to detect mild and severe cases of alcohol use and/or dependence (Ross & Tisdall, 1994). In addition, the CAGE scale has demonstrated comparable rates of sensitivity and specificity to that of larger scales, such as the 13-item Michigan Alcoholism Screening Test (MAST) (Hays et al., 1995).

The cut-off score for the CAGE scale has varied widely. The majority of studies use two "yes" answers to indicate a positive score (Mayfield et al., 1974; Beresford et al., 1990). Others interpret any affirmative response as an indicator of alcohol dependence (Ewing, 1984). The lower the cut-off score, the more sensitive and less specific the scale will become. When using a cut-off score of two or more, this scale demonstrates a sensitivity rate of 75–91 percent, and a specificity rate of 77–96 percent. These percentages change to a sensitivity rate of 60–100 percent, and a specificity rate of 78–88 percent when the cut-off point is decreased to one affirmative response. The cut-off score should be determined in response to the base rate of alcoholism in the environment of the subject group and in response to what the test is given to assess (Liskow & Campbell, 1995). This study would require a lower cut-off score (one "yes" response) in order to detect as many alcohol dependent people as possible. This form of detection will give a higher false positive rate, but it will also ensure that fewer alcoholics will go undetected and untreated.

The CAGE scale is not recommended for all clients. The CAGE scale should not be used with clients who have abstained from alcohol usage for two years prior to this assessment, nor those who are currently receiving or have received treatment for alcohol-related problems. The first group would be immune to detection by the scale, due to its concentration on the past year. The second group would require a more in-depth and specific assessment of their problem beyond the scope of the CAGE scale (Liskow & Campbell, 1995).

General Health Questionnaire (GHQ)

The GHQ (Goldberg, 1972) comes in a variety of forms, such as the 12-, 20-, 28-, 30-, and 60-item scale. Due to the fact that current society calls for the most rapid and accurate measure possible, the 12-item scale (GHQ-12) is the preferred version. The GHQ-12 can be completed in less than five minutes. This scale has been a valid indicator of probable general health cases, but it does not assess duration (Gureje & Obikoya, 1990). This allows the helping professional to detect a problem early, but does not indicate whether the problem is present on a regular basis. An example of this is that everyone gets depressed sometimes, but those who suffer from chronic depression would require more assistance than those caught in a temporary depression.

The GHQ-12 has been found to be an accurate measure of psychiatric morbidity in general medical and community settings (Gureje & Obikoya, 1990; Van Hemert et al., 1995). When using a cut-off score of 2/3, the sensitivity rate has been averaged at approximately 80 percent with a specificity rate of approximately 81 percent (Gureje & Obikoya, 1990; Kapur et al., 1984; Mari & Williams, 1985). While the 2/3 cut-off score is recommended, the 1/2 has also been used as a cut-off, yielding a 94 percent sensitivity rate, and a 62 percent specificity rate (Van Hemert et al., 1995). The GHQ-12 has been shown to be similar to the GHQ-60 and the GHQ-30 in its ability to detect psychiatric and psychosocial disorders.

It should be noted that Walter Hudson (1990) has developed a scale that could be more widely utilized to assess the same areas as the GHQ-12 as well as other areas of personal and social functioning. His scale is the Multi-Problem Screening Inventory (MPSI). While the MPSI has begun to receive some initial credence to its reliability and validity measures (Hudson & McMurtry, 1997), its 334 items limits its utilization. A computer-scoring program has been created for utilization with this scale that makes scoring the scale very rapid and provides a thorough and accurate in-depth assessment of client problems. However, this will not reduce the quantity of time needed for the client to complete this measure. If this scale could be compressed, but still maintain satisfactory reliability and validity measures, it could be applied to a multitude of settings. This scale, as well as Hudson's (1982) Global Screening Inventory (GSI) 25-item scale, which assesses a wide range of problem areas, is rated on a Likert scale. The problem is rated as experienced (1) none of the time, through (7) all of the time. This rating provides the evaluator with information on the severity of the problem, as well as its presence. Research on the reliability and validity of this measure, along with its applicability to practice settings would enhance its versatility in practice settings.

Diagnostic Assessment for Physical Ailments (DAPA)

The availability of a rapid assessment instrument capable of diagnosing physical ailments is nearly nonexistent. As a result, patients usually have to go through a series of repeating their symptoms first to the secretary in order to secure an appointment, then to the nurse who takes vital signs, and finally to the doctor who makes the final assessment. This repeated process can leave the patient feeling frustrated and anxious. Due to the inability to locate such a rapid assessment measure, the author created a measure called the Diagnostic Assessment for Physical Ailment (DAPA), which can be used in conjunction with the medical history form (filled out by all new patients) to assess changes in the patient's condition, and the location of these changes.

The DAPA scale was developed to assess a patient's physical symptoms and presenting problems. The values on the scale are: (1) Are you experiencing flu-like symptoms? (Coughing, a runny nose, swollen glands, nausea, or a fever); (2) Do you have a physical injury? (Broken or sprained bone, a muscle injury, a joint injury dislocation, a laceration, or a head injury); (3) Are you here to monitor or check up on a present or existing condition as a follow-up? (i.e. pregnancy, blood pressure, cholesterol level, allergies, diabetes, cancer, rectal or bladder dysfunction, ulcer, asthma, or skin irritation); (4) Are you here for a routine physical or immunization? (i.e. shots or vaccinations); (5) Are you experiencing sexual problems or dysfunctions?

These questions were created from a medical case history form as well as an adult and child medical assessment form. These questions were specifically created to deal with current problems because the client's medical history and incurring record should already detail past problems. Though the questions are broad, they are broken up into main topics to enable the physician to do a more focused assessment that targets the patient's presenting problem. This assessment tool combined with the alcohol and psychiatric assessment can provide a thorough and accurate assessment in a short amount of time. This combination of assessment instruments can also provide valuable information on the type of clinician needed by the client.

A growing concern is also for the rising number of older adults seeking medical attention. While a physician treats a physical crisis, the social worker can assess family and environmental concerns. Self-efficacy for older adults is important in relationship to their physical health as well. The more self-efficacious an older adult is the more health-promoting behaviors they will have as well as healthy outcomes (Elmore 2006; Greene & Sullivan, 2004).

Implications for Social Work Practice

Managed care does and will have a profound impact on the way that services are delivered, and on the duration of those services. While social workers may view these time limitations as a decrease in their role and ability to be effective, they should instead welcome the opportunity to become educated about empirically validated methods, and to utilize their assessment skills. The implementation of managed care has hindered social work provision of long-term service, but has enhanced social work effectiveness in screening and assessing client needs (Resnick & Tighe, 1997). Social workers can deal with the psychosocial and environmental aspects of illness. The link between mental health and somatic illness has become clear. Social workers have knowledge and training in the recognition and treatment of mental health problems that both medical specialists and physicians lack (Berkman, 1996).

Alternative treatment plans can also be used for those patients who require long-term treatment. Referrals for drug and alcohol programs or referrals to self help groups may strengthen the treatment due to shortened lengths of time a patient can be treated. Creativity is useful in finding good interventions with only limited amounts of time to work with the client (Gibelman & Mason, 2002).

Social Work Role

- Assess patient/client and family for ability to follow through on treatment plan
- Support client through assessment, diagnosis, treatment, rehabilitation, etc.
- Guide client through the system (what is covered, what is not, and to what extent)

- Educate and inform client and family members about the specific illness, coping techniques, outlook, etc.
- Address behavioral, emotional, or mental problems that may hinder decision making around the illness
- Identify, discuss, and obtain entitlement benefits
- Identify and facilitate linkages to appropriate non-medical resources (support groups, emergency food/housing, family/marital/couple/individual counseling, etc.)
- Share knowledge about the client and the family systems with the team to ensure their ability to effectively care for the client
- Advocate for patients who are dissatisfied with their care

Adapted from Berkman, 1996

- Contribute to research and policy evaluation

(Bachman et al., 2004)

Benefits

As elucidated in Chapter 1, social worker expertise and experience is still essential to social work practice, despite the role changes for social workers created by managed care. Critical to provision of coordinated care is the social worker's ability to assess and refer as appropriate to each branch of the interdisciplinary team. By flagging physiological ailments, the physician is saved from the task of screening the client/patient (Resnick & Tighe, 1997). By noting the client's psychosocial problems, the social worker enables the physician to deliver more comprehensive patient care (Berkman, 1996) and can determine when a patient's presenting problem is secondary to a mental health problem. Also, as previously noted, in addition to helping the physician to address the mental health needs of the client, social workers can also work within the primary care setting to address clients' environmental, psychosocial, and financial concerns, working with clients on family issues, financial and resource concerns, mental health issues, behavioral problems, medical noncompliance, etc. (Gross et al., 1983). Finally, also outlined in Chapter 1, the inclusion of social workers as members of the interdisciplinary team can also yield financial rewards to physicians, insurance providers, and other professionals on the team through the reduction of costs through early detection, early intervention, and decreased use/re-use of hospital services (Berkman, 1996; Law, 2006).

Social Work Education

In light of the changes that have, and will, take place as a result of the way services are paid for, the traditional social work educational programs must also alter their scope. Today's and tomorrow's social workers must be trained to work as members of interdisciplinary teams (Berkman, 1996). This training should include both benefits of the approach to clients, to the team itself, and to third party payers. Training such as this should facilitate a mutual respect and cooperation for the other disciplines and team members, as well as teach a clear sense of role. Support has grown for social work education to include a biomedical and psychological component. Social workers need to have knowledge of specific illness and diseases and their effect on other areas of functioning. Knowledge of the medical issues and ailments and an understanding of how they play out will assist the social worker in asking questions in order to assess the client. The social worker must be trained to work within this framework to address client problems in terms of prevention, eradication, and rehabilitation (Berkman, 1996). Social workers must also be educated in terms of brief and solution focused treatment, which will allow them to work within the time limitations, while maintaining effectiveness. Students of social work schools must be taught the importance of working from empirically supported treatment techniques. Utilizing an empirical foundation in practice will ensure both a funding and effectiveness of service delivery. This training should be provided through a variety of methods, including but not limited to, classroom lectures and discussions, practicums, field placements, and computerized simulation exercises.

Social workers have a major role to carry under the managed care model, but social workers must be flexible in adapting their skills in order to conform to this model. Social workers must utilize their skills in areas of assessment, diagnosis, referrals, and practice and program evaluations as part of an interdisciplinary team. There is an abundance of social work literature addressing the fit between professional values and managed care (Kane et al., 2003). The education for social workers must also be adapted to the role changes of the social work profession. The combination of the three proposed rapid assessment instruments allow social workers and other helping professionals the opportunity to work in collaboration to best serve the various needs of the clientele. According to Shera (1996), "managed care is here to stay, and social workers must rise to the challenge or let others take the lead" (p. 199).

Appendix: The CAGE and CAGEAID Questionnaires

The CAGE Questionnaires

- Have you ever felt you should *cut* down on your drinking?
- Have people *annoyed* you by criticizing your drinking? Have you felt bad or *guilty* about your drinking?

- Have you ever had a drink first thing in the morning to steady your nerves or get rid of a hangover *(eye-opener)*?

(*Source:* Mayfield et al., 1974)

The CAGE Questions Adapted to Include Drugs (CAGEAID)

- Have you felt you ought to cut down on your drinking or *drug use?*
- Have people annoyed you by criticizing your drinking or *drug use?*
- Have you felt bad or guilty about your drinking or *drug use?*
- Have you ever had a drink or *used drugs* first thing in the morning to steady your nerves or get rid of a hangover *or to get the day started?*

4 Development of Managed Information Systems for Human Services
A Practical Guide*

The twenty-first century can be characterized as the centerpiece of computer technology (Friedman, 2006). Clinicians and practitioners in human service agencies are thus participating in the transition to an "information society." The increased use of computers in the human services profession makes it necessary that practitioners and administrators become responsive to the computer aptitude. Social and political events have demonstrated the necessity of establishing human services based on data that provide rationale for planning and delivering services, evaluation of data, and fiscal support. Also, status indicators for the human services have changed as well. It will be rare if, in the future, social agencies do not incorporate computer use in their daily profession.

Agencies are finding that lack of resources no longer prevents the introduction of computers. However, as in all fields, the application of technology often lags behind its development. This chapter addresses the development and implementation of data management systems pertinent to helping agencies provide appropriate services to clients that are operating in a managed care context. The role of management information systems in managed care agencies is reviewed: managerial applications, client descriptive analyses, diagnosis, treatment planning, documentation of program implementation and effectiveness, research operations, specific clinical procedures, and educational functions. This chapter provides guidelines for establishing requisites for the development and selection of an adequate information system, the dissemination of information, and the application of relevant knowledge. Finally, the implications of management information systems for the field of social work are reviewed.

Basic Requisites

In designing an information system, the first requisite is its compatibility with other systems. Compatibility with other systems increases the information

* Chapter written with assistance of: Cyomara Fisher.

system's utility. For example, a client's needs in a mental health agency might be compared with that of a client's family service agency. A yearly evaluation of a management system should be conducted. The evaluation should address how the professionals use the system, what type of information is collected, and how the organization is structured to facilitate the use of data. Cetron et al., 1988 and Bell, 1973 (as cited in Mutschler & Jayaratne, 1994) found that a recent issue of Computer Utilization in Social Services (Spring 1990) contained a listing of fifty-four programs offering computerized clinical assessment, monitoring, and evaluation systems for social service practitioners.

An agency must address the following questions: What type of data is needed? What kind of software is required? What forms are required to collect this data? Who collects this data? How is the data stored? How is the confidentiality of the data to be insured? Is there a need for a data specialist? How can it be ensured that the appropriate individuals are involved in setting up the system and its subsequent use? Can the system be integrated with other systems agencies use?

The data collected in a human service agency should focus on the following phenomena: client and worker and treatment characteristics, and outcomes. Such data enable managed care to see, for example, how many clients were tested, what type of worker served the clients, and how many clients were seen. These data enhance an agency's ability to conduct cost-benefit analysis in order to determine how much a service unit costs. An information system should prove invaluable to the assessment of a client's treatment, the evaluation of services, the documentation of the intervention, and a follow-up.

Individuals developing the data system must determine how many files should be free-form in contrast to fixed-form format. Free-form records are used to document client assessments, treatments, and follow-ups. Such records are rich in descriptive information; however, they are difficult to condense and summarize. For example, if a practitioner wishes to view all the cases of potential suicides, the computer can be instructed to review all case documents and list cases where this potential was indicated. Yet, such analysis is slow and costly.

A fixed-form record specifies the exact nature of the data to be collected. A typical example would be a structured interview schedule to secure descriptive data on clients. The computer can quickly summarize the number of clients who received services during a particular period by their age, income, marital status, and number of children (Kreuger & Ruckdeschel, 1985).

Before an agency sets up an information system, as many workers as possible should be involved to enlist their support for the system's utilization. This involvement of the staff should take place at the earliest possible date. There should be joint decisions regarding the type of records needed. The agency must determine who will have access to the data and who will implement appropriate security measures to maintain the client's confidentiality. Securing a file is relatively simple with the technological developments in access coding.

Managerial Applications

The application of computer technology addresses a wide range of problems and administrative tasks. One major area of application in the delivery of services is the information management. Agencies are finding computers to be tremendous time savers in compiling service statistics, processing payrolls, billing for services, and preparing financial reports. Moreover, computer technology makes possible forms of inquiry previously inconceivable, particularly because the computer permits more timely expeditious use of sophisticated research techniques on routinely collected data.

Paper consumes an inordinate amount of time and energy in traditional human services agencies. The computer's word processing capability dramatically decreases paperwork in the production of reports, letters, memos, payrolls, tests, and forms. Once a draft of a document is written, there is a significant amount of time needed to modify the copy. Tailoring of different reports from the same store of information, outlining plans for worker development, and preparing budgets are other useful applications. Through word processing these functions can be quickly completed to facilitate operating in the managed care environment (Boyd et al., 1978).

Considering the present economy, computer applications can ease an agency's billing, financial screening procedures, the review and revision of fee schedules, the maintenance of accurate accounts of operating reserves to reduce cash-flow problems, and the documentation of services provided (Goplerud et al., 1985).

Client Descriptive Analyses

All agencies require a descriptive data to document whom they have served and how. These data provide a rationale for the agency budget and help in the planning for future needs. With appropriate intake forms, information is quickly and accurately gathered to determine (a) client to be served, (b) duration of service, (c) cost of service, (d) provider of the service, (e) follow-up results, and (f) additional service.

Dziegielewski (2004) found that every record must have basic information that includes the date and time of entry, interview notes that describe the client and the problem or situation that requires treatment, an assessment and initial treatment plan, and therapeutic objectives and treatment responses.

Thus, an agency can benefit from knowing who its clients are, which brings relevance to the data when approaching the sources of support and when gaining sanctions to extend the life of an agency. Once such a system is functional, an agency can conduct several cost-effectiveness analyses. This accountability requisite, evident in the 1980s, provides agencies with a means of deciding to alter, maintain, or expand services (Catherwood, 1974; Rapp, 1984).

Diagnosis, Treatment Planning, and Documentation of Program Implementation and Effectiveness

In the last decade, a number of scales have been developed to facilitate obtaining information necessary for workers to make adequate assessments of their clients (Howing et al., 1989; Newmark, 1985; Rittner & Wodarski, 1995). All inventories are computer scored to facilitate their use.

Comprehensive Screening Inventories

The Multiproblem Screening Inventory (MPSI) (Hudson, 1992) is a 334-item self-report scale that measures twenty-seven dimensions of family functioning. Subscales measure depression, self-esteem, partner problems, sexual discord, child problems, mother problems, personal stress, friend problems, neighbor problems, school problems, aggression, work associates, family problems, suicide, nonphysical abuse, physical abuse, fearfulness, ideas of reference, phobias, guilt, work problems, confused thinking, disturbing thoughts, memory loss, alcohol abuse, and drug abuse.

Questions are answered on a 7-point Likert scale (from "none of the time" to "all of the time"). This scale is computer scored to develop additional subscales. (Available from: WALMYR Publishing Co., P.O. Box 24779, Tempe, AZ 85285–4779). Table 4.1 lists other available Hudson scales.

The Family Assessment Screening Inventory (FASI) and the Multidimensional Adolescent Assessment Scale (MAAS) were designed to measure the degree of distinct and separate personal and social functioning problems in adolescent and adult populations. Furthermore, these are problem-focused social work assessment tools (Nugent et al., 2001).

Table 4.1 Other Hudson Scales

Child's Attitude toward Father	Index of Family Relations
Child's Attitude toward Mother	Index of Marital Satisfaction
Children's Behavior Rating Scale	Index of Parental Attitudes
Clinical Anxiety Scale	Index of Peer Relations
Computerized Scoring	Index of Self-Esteem
General Screening Inventory	Index of Sexual Satisfaction
Generalized Contentment Scale	Index of Sister Relations
The Global Screening Inventory	Nonphysical Abuse of Partner Scale
Index of Alcohol Involvement	Partner Abuse Scale: Nonphysical
Index of Attitudes toward	Partner Abuse Scale: Physical
Homosexuals	Physical Abuse of Partner Scale
Index of Brother Relations	Sexual Attitude Scale
Index of Clinical Stress	Index of Drug Involvement

Source: Hudson 1992

Hudson took subscales from the FASI that were deemed appropriate for use with adolescents and created the MAAS as an assessment scale for use with adolescent populations. Hudson's scales have been established as appropriate for research with adolescent and adult populations. The FASI produces information about twenty-five areas of personal and social functioning; they are: housing, physical safety, economic stress, nutrition and diet, family conflict, aggressive behavior, stress, family support, extended family, previous partners, community, employment, school, people outside family, alcohol use, drug use, domestic abuse, child abuse, extra-familial abuse, self-destructive behavior, childcare, parenting, psychological conditions, health conditions, and legal involvement; while the MAAS scores in sixteen areas which are: depression, self-esteem, mother problem, father problem, personal stress, friend problem, school problem, aggression, family problems, suicide, guilt, confused thinking, disturbing thoughts, memory loss, alcohol abuse, and drug abuse.

Scores on both measures produce a graph of the profile of the participant's problem status. This type of graph gives researchers and counselors an immediate picture of which respondents are having the most serious life problems (Faul & Hudson, 1997).

Other Relevant Scales

Many personalized computer systems now aid in the administration of more than fifty assessment inventories. These can provide a wealth of information on which clinicians can base their assessment of the client and can plan subsequent treatment (Hedlund et al., 1985). For example, National Computer Systems Professional Assessment Service (NCSPAS) has the capability to score assessment tests in the areas of (a) abnormal personality, (b) normal personality, (c) behavioral health and medicine, and (d) aptitudes and career/vocational interests. Table 4.2 lists other available NCSPAS tests.

By using the computer, practitioners can list goals, make progress notes, specify an intervention plan, and produce a timetable. It is possible to secure the documentation necessary to determine if the goals have been met by subsequently analyzing the data with respect to meeting the legal and administrative requisites (Carlson, 1985; Meldman et al., 1977). The amount of information provided by a computer analysis of the Minnesota Multiphasic Personality Inventory (MMPI) can truly facilitate the adoption of the scientific practitioner model (Hudson, 1992; Wodarski, 1986).

Research Operations

For research, computers are essential. Once information is organized and placed into the computer, complicated calculations become effortless routines: transformation of data, simple graphing of clients goals, and modification of data for further analysis made easier. The frequently used SPSS and other

Table 4.2 Other Available NCSPAS Tests

Adjective Checklist	Minnesota Multiphasic Personality
Bender Visual Motor Gestalt Test	Inventory (MMPI) Basic Service
California Psychological Inventory	MMPI-The Minnesota Report:
Career Assessment Inventory	Adult Clinical System
Clinical Analysis Questionnaire	MMPI-The Minnesota Report:
The Exner Report for the Rorschach	Personnel Selection System
Comprehensive System	Multidimensional Personality
General Aptitude Test Battery	Questionnaire
Giannetti Online Psychosocial	Myers-Briggs Type Indicator
History	The Rorschach Comprehensive System
Guilford-Zimmerman Temperament	Self-Description Inventory
Survey	Sixteen Personality Factors
Hogan Personality Inventory	Questionnaire
Million Adolescent Personality	Strong-Campbell Interest Inventory
Inventory-Clinical	Temperament and Values Inventory
Million Adolescent Personality	Vocational Information Profile
Inventory-Guidance	Word and Number Assessment
Million Behavioral Health Inventory	Inventory

statistical packages are now available for personal desktop computers (Butler, 1986). This innovation increases the capability of practitioners to execute basic statistical analyses on their cases. Thus, the ability to analyze different practice phenomena is enhanced. However, as with all technology, an adequate conceptual plan should guide the selection of appropriate analyses.

Development of Management Information Systems

In summary, computers can assist human service workers in attaining the following clinical research goals:

1. Administration and scoring of tests
2. Interpretation and reporting:

   (a) Wechsler
   (b) Rorschach
   (c) MMPI

3. Client program planning and evaluation

   (a) goals
   (b) case progress
   (c) intervention plan

   (d) timetable
   (e) document referral process

4. Program documentation

   (a) data recording and illustration
   (b) data analysis
   (c) attainment of legal and administrative requisites

5. Research applications

   (a) client progress
   (b) calculations
   (c) transformation of data
   (d) graphing client and administrative variables
   (e) updating information in a database

Specific Practice Procedures that Can Be Computerized

There are numerous concrete items that are easily computerized regardless of the practice context. Contracts formulated between client and workers can be checked for the inclusion of the following: purposes of the interaction, targeted problems and areas of difficulties to be worked on, various goals and objectives to be accomplished, client and therapist duties, delineation of administrative procedures, techniques to be used, duration of contracts and criteria for termination, renegotiation procedures and referrals (Wodarski & Bagarozzi, 1979).

Agencies can use goal-setting forms that specify a client's problem, plans for therapy, short- and long-term goals, and plans for termination, follow-up procedures, and so forth. These forms facilitate the evaluation of clients' progress in meeting their treatment goals. Additionally, a summary form specifies the overall treatment plan, including termination and follow-up procedures. Access to this documentation should improve the services offered to clients.

Other computer functions to improve evaluation include checking to see if practice notes summarizing the major events of the client's last visit are recorded within a reasonable time, such as 72 hours after the session, and determining whether the follow-up visits are executed when necessary and placed in the client's record within a reasonable time. Also to be included are a letter to all third parties regarding treatment plans and diagnosis, summary termination notes and follow-up procedures, and, if necessary, a letter to the referring professional or family doctor regarding the termination of services, all within one week of closing a case. In all instances, the energy and the time necessary to complete the forms should be kept to a minimum (Rinn & Vernon, 1975). Computers facilitate the execution of these requisite clinical tasks, by simplifying the record-keeping process.

Educational Functions

Through the use of educational programs, computers can help in preparing the beginning practitioner to work with clients. Before working with parents who abuse their children, the worker might be trained to assess adequately marital interaction, child management practices, and social and vocational satisfaction, and to implement the appropriate intervention strategies according to the assessment (Ruggiero et al., 2006).

To assess the worker's theoretical accuracy, an objective examination or assessment battery—for example, on task-centered casework, family therapy or behavioral social work—can be given. Once workers achieve acceptable scores on an assessment battery, they can then move on to implementing interventions based on the theoretical framework.

Practice skill levels can be determined by asking the worker to review a contrived case, to make a diagnosis, to design an intervention plan, and to describe the success of the plan to the satisfaction of practitioners who have already demonstrated their competencies. Education exercises can be programmed and computed to help the practitioner acquire competencies through repeated exercises.

Simulation

Simulation technologies are defined rather consistently throughout the literature simply as an operating model of a real system; that is, physical representations of reality (Cash, 1983). Simulation is a category within the general class of scientific tools known as models. Models are certain ways of representing reality, and students can compare the simulated experience to what they believe and experience in the real world (Wodarski et al., 1996). Simulations are often used to promote participatory learning through acting out lifelike situations, thus allowing simulation participants to gain an understanding of problems they may encounter in their practice and encouraging a new perspective and problem-solving framework. Well-designed simulations allow serendipitous, incidental learning as well as achievement of planned learning objectives.

There are many practical uses for simulations in the classroom setting. Theory can be applied immediately. Simulations can be used to break the ice, impart facts (though rarely used for this purpose alone), develop empathic sensitivity and values clarification, examine dimensions and dynamics of social problems, explore the future, and refine and immediately apply analytical research skills (Shay, 1980). Moreover, simulations heighten interest, change attitudes, facilitate skills acquisition, and assist in cognitive learning and personal growth (Faherty, 1983). Conclusive evidence, however, is available only for heightened interest. In skills acquisition, there is evidence to show that simulations aid in the integrative thought process (Shay, 1980).

One clear advantage simulation has over learning in real life situations is that the student is protected from the consequences of error in a real system. That is, practice skills can develop without negative consequences to a client. Another advantage of simulation over live practice is that in the early stages of training, stress can be removed and then replaced when the skill has been mastered (Lewis & Gibson, 1977).

As with any technology, however, there are several disadvantages to using simulation technologies in social work education. First, simulations are unpredictable; they only benefit certain students some of the time. There is also a lack of instructor control in many simulations. There can be a great investment of time, energy, and monetary costs in carrying out a simulation. Finally, there is a struggle between simplicity and complexity: simple simulations are easier to use but are of less educational value, and complex simulations are too difficult to use. Despite limitations, however, the strengths of simulations outweigh their weaknesses.

Given the advantages and disadvantages of simulation use, when does one choose to do a simulation? The decision might be based on the following criteria: will a simulation create a situation likely to be encountered in real life? will it help prepare the practitioner to deal with ambiguities and complexities found later in life? The application of simulations is relatively unexplored. Only creativity limits the use of this teaching medium. Simulations integrate theory and practice.

For a simulation experience to be effective on any level, it must be relevant and have sound internal pedagogical elements and processes (appropriate learning objectives, related to and complementing lecture, self-reflection, and relevant student exercises). It must also facilitate achievement of specific learning objectives. The literature also suggests that the simulation experience heightens interest in the learning experience. This is especially true when the simulation is a computer simulation (Phillips, 1984a).

Types of Models

Different simulation model typologies are found in the literature. One useful typology classifies simulations as "person models," "person-machine models," or "pure machine models." The person model employs only human decision makers. These are usually simple or structured role-plays, behavior games, sensitivity experiences, and many types of skills training. These simulations will not be reviewed in this book due to the extensive existing reviews in the literature. The person-machine model makes use of the interaction of a person with a machine, usually a computer. New computer technologies make this the most exciting area to pursue in social work education. The third type of simulation is the pure machine model. These simulations include problem solving by machines and are pure mathematical models of reality. Their promise for human services has not yet been explored.

Person-Machine Model

A person-machine model (e.g., computer simulation) employs a high degree of abstraction from reality. In computer simulations, all of the features of a real system are reduced to logical decision rules and operations, which are then programmed for computer manipulation (Meinert, 1972).

Computer technology is blossoming at a staggering rate. In fact, the computer is becoming so important that unless students become familiar with this machine, the student is destined to be unsuccessful in both school and the workplace (Green, 1984). Hence, it is imperative that computer interaction be required in the education of a social worker.

In discussing the utility of computer simulations for social work research, Fuller asserts that computer technology is now within the range of almost every practicing social worker (Fuller, 1970). Access to a computer and programming is as near as the extension service of a university's computer center. Even so, the literature regarding direct application of this technology on the social service agency and practitioner levels remains sparse (Wodarski, 1986).

The computer entered the counseling profession in the early 1960s, with practitioners exploring the use of technology in counseling. Throughout the 1960s and into the 1970s the computer was seen as an assistant to the counselor, and programs were developed that taught problem-solving skills and provided information. By 1970, two annotated bibliographies and two small volumes were written on computer technology in counseling professions. Recently, informational and diagnostic databases have been developed, and models of systematic interventions, mechanical clients with which to practice and supervisory monitoring systems have all come into existence (Phillips, 1984a). As the use of the computer continues to make breakthroughs into the helping professions, the educational value of the computer also increases.

The computer has inherent value for education, which gives it a separate productive purpose that will coexist with its operating functions in the work place. Phillips discusses the attractiveness of computers for education in the tasks and methods of the individual's instruction (Phillips, 1984a). It can be seen as an intelligent tutor, thus reducing the student-teacher ratio. Fascination with the medium is a plus; it may induce longer study time and greater learning. There are two ways by which a computer can help a trainee with skills acquisition. First, there is didactic presentation with example of a skill, and there is simulation (Phillips, 1984b). Its use as a simulator has been compared to that of a cadaver for surgeons.

Self-Help Programs

Programs are now being written for the general public that can be used or adapted for social work education (Chamberlin, 2005). These programs are called "life enrichment software" or "psyche ware programs" which are designed to accept decision responses from one or more people. The programs allow multiple branching sequences. Programs include Eliza, who simulates a nondirective therapist; Mind Prober, which estimates another person's attitudes; Child Pace and Discover Your Baby, which produces improved parenting; and Coping with Stress and the Party, which teaches the adolescent about the effects of alcohol. Finally, Skip is a highly interactive program that allows users to learn about aspects of their own personality. According to White, there are enormous possibilities for computers in therapist education (White, 1984). There is also a danger, however, to the general public in these "self-help" programs. White compares them to the "self-awareness groups" of the 1960s. Hence, it is important that social workers be familiar with these types of programs (Parker-Oliver & Demiris, 2006).

Simulated Counselor

Programs must be interactive in order to be used effectively for social work education. Interactive programs have multiple branching-out contingencies that depend on the responses of the user. To be effective, the computer must be able to understand the client's natural language. The program also must be able to follow a therapeutic plan when dealing with a client. This can be problematic, but inroads into research on artificial language have been made. Eliza, for example, simulates a nondirective therapist; it analyzes each statement typed into the computer and then responds with a question or comment. This program is limited because it cannot recognize nonsense and it lacks intuition.

Morton is a computer-assisted therapy program that deals with the shortcomings of Eliza. Morton attends to depression and a related, specific psychological problem that has particular treatment strategies using a variety of cognitive and behavioral therapeutic techniques. This program uses multiple-choice items and case vignettes to aid the user in identifying dysfunctional thoughts. It deals with those thoughts that are assumed to be the major source of depression (Wagman & Kerber, 1984). Another interaction program, PLATO Dilemma Counseling System (PLATO DCS), is designed for the treatment of avoidance problems. It teaches dilemma counseling and solves specific problems. Because these programs must be exact, trainees learn to be precise throughout the therapeutic process. The programs facilitate learning and are patient, reliable, and efficient. Trainees can also experience what their future clients may feel like by using the systems.

Simulated Clients

The previous programs all take on the role of the therapist. These simulations are helpful in teaching exactly "how to." However, there are other programs that simulate a client and allow trainees to practice their skills. One such program, as described by Lichtenberg, is INTERACT (Lichtenberg et al., 1984). The assumption behind this program is that counseling is social interaction: It consists of a series of verbal and/or nonverbal exchanges. The INTERACT program analyzes the counselor-client transactions or response contingencies. It helps trainees learn how to obtain certain classes of responses that have been shown to contribute to favorable counseling outcomes. INTERACT also develops an awareness of the impact of those responses on their clients and the effects of their clients on their production of those responses.

A fascinating program described by Lichtenberg et al. is CLIENT 1 (1984). This is an interactive computer simulation of client behavior in an initial client interview. The model client is a 30-year old who is verbal, motivated, and not overly resistant. The client can talk about several topics but they are not of equal importance; only one is his primary concern. Each topic is ranked from general to specific, and each statement is ranked according to threat value. The counselor's task is to move the client toward verbalization of a specific and threatening statement of his or her problem. Progress is defined as moving toward specificity and threat. The computer continually re-evaluates the strength of the counseling relationship, and the level of trust. It is determined by the accuracy and appropriateness of the counselor's response. If the trainee is consistently inaccurate or inappropriate, a low "good counselor average" will occur and the session will be prematurely terminated.

Simulated client programs have many uses in social work education. They are flexible and allow a changing of variables and they can be used over and over again. CLIENT 1 is consistent and durable, and it will allow recognition of negative counseling habits. Counseling skills can be broken down into parts, and reflection on their use is possible. The clients can be made simple or complex, and they will not be harmed by the trainee's mistakes. This will allow the trainee to see the value in simply reflecting until good data are available. Finally, the trainee can move back to any portion of the interview and play "what if I had said . . ." This option, which can be invaluable, is not available on any other training medium.

Video Technology

Video technology represents a combination of the person-model and the person-machine model. It can belong to either category depending upon its use. For instance, it can be used in conjunction with computer simulation, or it can be used as a way to confront one's own performance in a role-play process. Self-observation is the most frequent application.

Observation of oneself on videotape can be very beneficial to skill acquisition. For example, Hosford and Johnson (1983) performed an experiment on teaching techniques using video playback. They found that using "self-as-a-model" reduced almost all inappropriate behaviors by approximately 100 percent. Observation of self also helped improve performance, especially if feedback was provided by a supervisor or teacher. However, confrontation of one's image on tape can be anxiety-producing for some people and may actually block learning. Thus, positive feedback is necessary.

Videodisc Simulation

In making the transition from informal simulations to laboratory modeling simulations, remember that this text discusses phases of development rather than distinct conceptual categories. The transition to what the literature refers to as "laboratory simulation" seems to indicate an increase in structure or structured task, which the earlier informal simulations lacked.

As technology has become more sophisticated and people have begun to be more creative, many new educational tools have become available. Interactive video is one such tool. Iuppa defines interactive video as any video system in which the sequence and selection of messages is determined by the user's response to the material presented (1984). There are computer languages and software packages that will allow a person who knows absolutely nothing about programming languages to create an interactive simulation (Hosie & Smith, 1984).

Interactive video requires the use of a video cassette recorder or a videodisc. The former are cumbersome and not very practical. Since they do not have random access to any segment of the recorded material as the disks do, video cassettes are too slow. With the videodisc's greater sophistication, there is not much in the way of coursework that could not be converted into a computer-controlled interactive videodisc (Pribble, 1985). For example, the Interactive Technology Groups, based in Sante Fe, New Mexico, has developed a five-disc course on human relation skills. Hence, a beginning has been made into this exciting and promising field (Pribble, 1985).

The videodiscs allow fast and random access to any part of the disc in less than a second. The discs hold up to 54,000 single video frames per side and can accommodate up to 30 minutes of moving imagery. Of course, the microcomputer controls the access, evaluates responses (as in the CLIENT 1 program), displays text, and even asks questions. Hence, the trainee can learn verbal and nonverbal skills before working with actual clients. The experience of video simulation should include as much video presentation of real images as possible. Interactive video allows trainees to see the consequences of their choices and this is the real strength of this type of learning medium.

Videodisc training systems are not only for training the social worker, but also for keeping records concurrent for post analysis research. These systems combine the technology of programmed instruction, curriculum-building, computer control for customized instruction and management of instruction, and the enormous capability for storage and random-access retrieval of image, sound, and textual information inherent in the videodisc. While the current development costs are still very high, these systems offer enormous potential for keeping service staffs current with the explosion in rules, regulations, practices, and knowledge, and for preparing clients for service by providing background information, sensitization to issues, and such (Geiss & Viswanathan, 1986).

There is some evidence of the effectiveness of videodisc training (Pribble, 1985). In 1984, the University of West Florida trained a group of welfare department employees in the administration of food stamps using a 16-hr interactive videodisc course. The trainees finished the training course 25 percent faster than that of the control group, which was taught in the traditional manner. Also, 66 percent of the interactive group passed the post test, while only 50 percent of the control group passed the post test.

An authoring system for interactive computer simulations is available and can be adapted to simulations in social work education. The hardware and software of the authoring system was developed by the staff of the Interactive Videodisc for Special Education Technology (IVSET). IVSET had five criteria in developing their authoring system for the education of children with developmental disabilities. The programmer should be able to use the system regardless of computer experience, and flexibility of instruction is recommended. The system should collect data to analyze. A teacher should be able to author a program. Finally, the system should be capable of summarizing student data and monitoring student's progress.

Informational Requisites

The first requisite in developing an information management system is to determine how the data will be collected and what forms are necessary. It is essential that the collected data be reliable and valid.

Second, it is essential that the agency consider the number of files that will be necessary for the collection of these data. The more files that are needed, the more complicated and costly a management information system becomes. The files should also be evaluated for how much data they will contain, how they will interface with other systems, and whether the central processing unit can handle the numbers.

Selecting a Management Information System

The design of a management information system entails specifying an agency's needs and the purpose of the system. An assessment of financial and time resources is the next step, followed by a review of an agency's needs and the resources provided by those knowledgeable about information systems. If available, a number of different management systems should be studied.

Second, consult various experts and others working with the system to see what they are doing with them. Visit a similar agency in which an information system is already operational; pilot test the system before full-scale implementation. Also, read journals that have sections devoted to the latest computer applications to human service agencies (i.e., The Behavior Therapist by the Association of the Advancement of Behavior Therapy). Finally, after selection and implementation, it is necessary to annually review the system to make modifications and improvements as needed. Systems should be designed and integrated with other systems. This permits analysis across system data systems.

The Dissemination of Information and Application of Relevant Knowledge

Practitioners are to participate in management information systems research, which is a necessary condition in developing the treatment technology needed for the field; schools of social work must begin to teach the skills required. The ability to formulate questions, choose the data options needed to answer these questions, and make rational decisions based on the data—not on the vague criteria presently employed—is critical.

Another challenge will be implementing effective technologies as they are developed. Using a rational method for choosing change strategies to meet client needs should be a primary function of research in social work. In an area where tradition, authority, and "common sense" practice have ruled for years, a "database" set of alternatives should facilitate the effective delivery of services. It would be a mistake, however, to assume that the availability of good empirical research will lead automatically to improved services. The history of knowledge utilization in other human services fields shows clearly that the change process is much more complicated than is implied by a simple linear model, which suggests that the productions of knowledge leads naturally to its utilization. In fact, in most cases, the effective dissemination and use of new findings are as difficult as their production (Hartmann et al., 1981).

The problem of knowledge utilization can be seen as an adoption problem related to the issue of how to train practitioners to search for and evaluate research data when choosing intervention alternatives. In certain cases, practitioners may be capable of conducting their own evaluation, but in most cases, they must rely on information and conclusions reported by more qualified professional researchers and evaluators. Certainly, social workers should be trained to personally monitor the effects of their intervention, gather feedback on the direction and magnitude of change, interpret studies for their relevance, and implement time-series designs. But workers rarely possess the resources and skills of a professional evaluator which are necessary to perform a summary evaluation of the effects of a program or a change strategy (Tornatzky et al., 1983; Wodarski, 1981).

Even after practitioners are exposed to new techniques and show that they are employing aspects of a new treatment, evaluations suggest that they are practicing in the same manner as in the past but have merely labeled this activity differently (Mullen & Dumpson, 1972). Thus, to ensure that professionals are kept abreast of current treatment developments, and will implement them, the incentive structure of social work practice will be changed. Social workers will have to be rewarded.

Issues for the Field

First, preparing human service workers to use computers in helping clients is essential. Even if information management systems become readily available and agencies implement them, technical expertise will be necessary to aid in the interpretation and summarization of the knowledge they produce. Moreover, experts should be prepared to summarize the data and disseminate them to other agencies that deal with similar clients. This process will add to the knowledge base of service providers. In the absence of such integration, chaos may ensue.

Second, yearly evaluations are required to update a data system as needed. Sufficient time should be spent in setting up an adequate system, since it is much more difficult and costly to change a data system once it is operational.

Third, the human service field must come to grips with defining outcomes and standards for service. When outcomes are ambiguous, standardizing them is impossible and comparisons across agencies are meaningless. Information systems can be utilized to plan and implement agency goals. For example, computers can (a) facilitate an empirical approach to the identification, collection, organization, and analysis of data and information about clients; (b) aid in the study of the component processes and outcomes of human service delivery systems; (c) clarify the state of human service needs and how practitioners can facilitate the strengths of clients; (d) aid in practitioners' learning theories and practicing various skills; and (e) facilitate the evaluation of different theories of behavioral change and intervention.

In essence, for informational management systems to facilitate the provision of relevant services to clients, the following recommendations are proposed: the field should develop standards for practice, data management systems should be developed so that human service agencies can interact with one another, such as mental health interfacing with criminal justice and child welfare programs, and at the national level, a data system might be developed which would lead to the identification of how social policies of both federal and state governments affect clients.

The client change process and the interventions used to help clients are complex. Computers can facilitate an understanding of these processes, and thus enhance a practitioner's ability to tailor appropriate interventions built on a client's strengths.

5 Psychosocial Treatment Configurations*

Introduction

Psychosocial treatments that work with clients in a multimodal and a multilevel configuration can be both more involved and more time consuming, as well as oftentimes more comprehensively effective. Pressures and demands on the field of social work and social workers to meet the disparate needs of a rapidly changing client base within an even more rapidly changing culture and social system are at an all time high. The emphasis on effective and rapid interventions is acute. There is no perfect answer to this situation. At best, it will be managed through the slow progress of trial and error from the dedicated patience and perseverance of this field's professionals.

Certainly one of the most influential factors pressuring the field is the requirements of managed care. This is easily seen as the unflinching demand for evidence based outcome treatment procedures that can be utilized within a relatively short time frame. There is a feeling of urgency to find the briefest treatment methods possible that can be readily generalized to fit broad categorical definitions of client needs. Contrast this urgency with the needs of a client seeking help from a social worker, to find within his or her therapeutic relationship, a caring, relaxed, and personable supporter whom they can trust to treat them with respect and unrushed empathy.

Add to this conflict of contrasting needs between the system and the consumer the fact that the lives and problems of clients are increasingly complex. Modern culture brings up many more interpersonal problems than it ever begins to answer, leaving people needing direction and connection to resources and solutions. Thyer (2001) states that the social work profession suffers from a dearth of empirically based studies of practice outcomes and should consider itself more an applied profession that finds solutions to psychosocial problems.

Increased attention is being placed on the need for practioners to be aware of things happening in other branches of science. Integrated therapies (matrix therapies) that may call for utilizing new pharmacological developments are being used with more regularity in areas such as addiction and mental health (Vaughn & Howard, 2004). As well as awareness for developing

---

*   Chapter written with the assistance of: Stephen Nicholson.

modalities, practitioners must also be sensitive to the type and depth of interventions being used. Just for example a sense of self-efficacy can be crucial in dealing with trauma (Benight & Bandura, 2004). There is great need for the appropriate use of the most effective methods for a particular circumstance. A significant report (Bloom et al., 2001: 1513) addressing the psychosocial needs of women with breast cancer states:

> There is evidence to indicate the best model of therapy for particular clinical settings, but many therapies have much in common (Tapper, 1999). For example, evidence from meta-analyses of randomized controlled trials indicates the efficacy of supportive and cognitive—behavioral therapies in the treatment of depressive disorders in women with breast cancer (Devine & Westlake, 1995; Sheard & Maguire, 1996) and the efficacy of individual and group therapies (Sheard & Maguire). It may be that the features of therapy common to all psychological interventions, such as an empathic manner, listening, affirmation, reassurance, and support, generate the observed outcome. Certain women are more comfortable with the privacy of individual counseling; other women benefit from group counseling, where they share the commonality of their experience with group members (Fawzy & Fawzy, 1998). Good support from family and friends is a protective factor, and lack of support may be associated with poorer emotional adjustment (Bloom, Stewart, Johnston, Banks, & Fobair, 2001; Roberts et al., 1994; Zemor & Shepel, 1989). The evidence supporting the provision of psychosocial care to women with breast cancer is clear. The challenge for the social work profession is to ensure that women can obtain appropriate help when needed.

Psychosocial Treatment Configuration

The role of the social worker in the evolving managed health care system must address the foci that formulate the empirical basis of practice. Newer methods of meta-analysis are identifying whether interventions are proving efficacious in meeting client needs and what interventions are working best in which situations, e.g., Shadish & Baldwin's (2003) article on meta-analysis of marriage and family therapy interventions in which its efficacy was verified. The various foci for evidence-based practice are elucidated as follows: worker and client characteristics, components of treatment, the type of context, level of intervention and relapse-prevention procedures. Substantial volumes of studies support psychosocial intervention. Only selected and classic studies are mentioned here to illustrate the points.

Worker and client characteristics. A number of worker variables, such as social class, race and ethnicity, religion, age, sex, and verbal skills, have been related to therapeutic outcome research (Harrison et al. 1992; Wodarski, 1997). For example, Faver (2004) presented findings from a study of fifty female service providers and social reformers that focused on relational spirituality. It was revealed that the women caregivers were sustained by being relationally connected to various aspects of their lives, including a sacred source of love and strength. This is also a characteristic that could be matched to some client perspectives of life.

One practice generalization taken from the literature is that differences between clients and workers should be minimal. The data point to a homogeneous grouping of workers and clients on various characteristics (Garfield & Bergin, 1986; Gurman & Razin, 1977; Hilarski & Wodarski, 2001). Harrison, Wodarski, and Thyer (in press) suggest that client and therapist be matched on such characteristics as age, sex, race and ethnicity, values, attitudes, and socioeconomic status. However, research also indicates that practical experience reduces the significance of this relationship (Durlak, 1979). Until more studies are conducted to delineate exact parameters of these practice interactions, it is recommended that inexperienced practitioners work with clients who are similar to themselves on relative attributes. Support of this proposition is derived also from literature on attraction that indicates that similarity between worker and client on certain variables increases the attractiveness of the therapeutic context, thus increasing the probability that the clients would remain in therapy, a necessary condition for behavior change (Shapiro, 1974; Yutrzenka, 1995).

Professionals versus Paraprofessionals. Earlier studies that evaluated services offered by professionals as compared to those offered by paraprofessionals have found that professionals did not necessarily give better service (Durlak, 1979; Emrick et al., 1977). These studies, and more recent ones, suggest that the reason paraprofessionals do as well as, or better than, professionals may revolve around their being closer to their clients on various attributes, thus enabling clients to identify with the worker, place more trust in him or her, and feel less alienation (Beutler & Kendall, 1995; Stein & Lambert, 1995). Research has shown consistently that workers who exhibit warmth, accurate empathetic understanding, and genuineness lay the foundation for effective therapeutic outcome. These characteristics may be the common elements that consistently set up and contribute to successful interventions.

However, research findings show that after graduation only a third of the professionally trained social workers possess acceptable levels of such qualities as warmth and empathy (Wodarski et al., 1988; Wodarski et al., 1995). The relationship between these attributes and professional education is not clear (Garfield, 1971).

Worker Characteristics: Practice Recommendations. A number of researchers have studied worker variables and their relationship to therapeutic outcome. Many variables are mentioned in repeated studies and are substantiated. The literature is conclusive and should be applied to the training of workers. Thus, the following empirically based statements can be made regarding worker variables and their influence on practice.

1. Client and worker should be grouped according to similar attributes to facilitate the attractiveness of the worker. Extreme differences should be avoided. The matching for beginning practitioners is necessary to isolate the goodness of fit between the inexperienced worker and the appropriate client.
2. All workers should possess acceptable levels of empathy, warmth, and genuineness.
3. Practitioners should exhibit credibility and show acceptance of the client through being personable. They should possess the ability to provide support and structure and to create the expectation that the therapeutic process will produce desired changes.

The list below summarizes the common factors of the effective worker based on the aggregate of replicated studies are summarized below (Shealy, 1995).

Common Factors of Worker Efficacy

- Congruency
- Acceptance/Unconditional Positive Regard
- Empathy
- Understanding/Communicate Understanding
- Encourage Autonomy; Responsibility
- Ability to Relate/Develop Alliance
- Well-Adjusted
- Interested in Helping
- Provide Treatment as Intended
- Exploration of Client
- Expectation for Improvement
- Emotionally Stimulating/Challenging/Not Afraid of Confrontation
- Firm, Direct; Can Set Limits
- Work Hard for Client/Persistent
- Nurturing

Treatment Components

Length of Therapy. A substantial number of evaluated studies has been produced in the last three decades that have a profound impact on traditional therapeutic practice. Major changes have come about because of these studies; one in particular being the length of therapy (Fischer, 1978; Shefler et al., 1995). In the past, therapy was considered a long involved process. Current trends, however, indicate that the optimal number of outpatient service visits is between 8 and 16, with the maximum being 20. Inpatient services should consist of 10, 21, or 30 days. Current research indicates that brief directive interventions have a consistent outcome advantage in the treatment of a multitude of disorders (Giles et al., 1993). Reid (1978), Stuart (1974), and others provide a rationale for the development of a short-term model of therapy for social work practice. Moreover, managed health care will support only payment for empirically based treatment that is of short duration, the rationale being that more evidence supports short-term care except for a few significant chemical problems (Johnstone et. al., 1995; Nickelson, 1995).

Behavior Acquisition. A second new major focus involves helping clients learn new behaviors to deal with their specific situations (Wodarski and Wodarski, 1993). This emphasis is in opposition to that of changing attitudes or motivation first and positing that behavior change should follow. Research evidence is accumulating to indicate that if clients are taught behaviors that enable them to influence their external and internal environments (e.g., self-management procedures, appropriate assertive behavior, and problem solving), their social functioning increases.

Development of behaviors is believed to occur optimally in structured therapeutic contexts; that is, where intervention procedures follow a sequential pattern to develop and maintain socially relevant behaviors. Such patterns usually consist of mutually agreed upon contracts that include goals, methods, termination criteria, and the rights and responsibilities of client and worker.

Empirically Supported Interventions. According to Thyer & Wodarski (1998) the development of psychosocial treatments which have been shown through credible scientific tests to really be of help to clients provides an exciting arena for social work practice. Perhaps not to every client with a particular difficulty, and perhaps not to the point of complete resolution or cure, but for many problems we are in a position to offer professional social work services which are quite likely to benefit a significant proportion of clients with a certain problem, to a clinically meaningful extent. The American Psychiatric Association (e.g. APA, 1995), The American Psychological Association (APA, 1995; Chambless, 1996), and the National Association of Social Workers (NASW) are busy at work developing practice guidelines which contain guidance as to what treatments are first indicated for particular problems. Within the American Psychological Association, careful compilations are being made of psychosocial interventions that work for particular disorders (see Sanderson & Woody, 1995), and this information will be having an increasing influence on the conduct of practice.

Within all human services, it is coming increasingly evident that certain psychosocial treatments are effective for particular problems and some are not. In one study of relapse prevention, men and women responded differently to the same treatment (Csiernick & Troller, 2002). A number of books summarize these findings, such as Giles (1993), Ammerman et al. (1993), and the Institute of Medicine (1989), as do some recent articles within social work, notably Gorey (1996), MacDonald, Sheldon & Gillespie (1992), Rubin (1985), Thomlison (1984), Thyer (1995a), Gorey et al. (1996) and Reid & Hanrahan (1982). Contrary to the nihilistic view that "virtually any intervention can be justified on the grounds that it has as much support as alternative methods" (Witkin, 1991, p. 158), numerous outcome studies comparing various forms of psychosocial treatment regularly find that certain types of interventions work better than others for particular problems. Consult any recent issues of *Research on Social Work Practice*, the *Journal of Consulting and Clinical Psychology*, or *Archives of General Psychiatry* for evidence of this contention. Also various alternative or nontraditional approaches are being looked at more seriously (Arnold, 1995).

Empirically based treatment technologies consist of behavioral approaches to the solution of interpersonal problems. Numerous data based behavioral technologies are available for workers to use in assessment and helping clients acquire necessary behaviors to operate in their environments. For example Matto (2001) determined that the Draw-A-Person: Screening Procedure for Emotional Disturbance was an accurate predictor of behavior in children aged 6–12 yrs.

Every year there is more data supporting the successful history of behavior modification practice with children classified as hyperactive, autistic, delinquent, and retarded, and adults classified as antisocial, retarded, neurotic, and psychotic (Anderson-Butcher et al., 2003; Davidson & Neale, 1994; Glass & Arnkoff, 1992; Goldfried et al., 1990; Mrug et al., 2001; Thyer, 1995b). The technologies with accumulating empirical history are:

- Relaxation Training
- Assertiveness Training
- Anger Management
- Stress Management
- Problem-solving Skills
- Self-esteem Building
- Urge Control
- Relapse Prevention
- Eye Movement Desensitization and Reprocessing (EMDR)
- Mindfulness-based Cognitive Therapy

The following is a categorization of the areas of possible application of behavioral technology in social work practice according to treatment context. The majority of approaches could be used by the behavioral health social worker. Each application has substantial empirical support. A further elaboration of theory, research, and illustrations of the application of the techniques is available in Wodarski & Bagarozzi (1979) and Thyer & Wodarski (2007).

Treatment Context

Children. (For extensive discussion, see Dulmus & Wodarski, 1996.)

1. *Foster care.* Development of behavioral management programs and appropriate parenting skills for both natural and foster parents. Training parents to use contingency contracts, stimulus control, and time-out

procedures to facilitate their children's development of social skills needed for effective adult functioning.

2. *Schools.* Helping to decrease absenteeism; increasing appropriate academic behavior, such as reading comprehension, vocabulary development, and computation skills; increasing interpersonal skills, such as the ability to share and cooperate with other children and adults; and decreasing disruptive behaviors.

3. *Juvenile Courts.* Helping decrease deviant behavior and increase prosocial behavior by contingency contracting; programming significant adults to provide reinforcement for pro social behavior; and developing programs for training children in those behavioral skills that will allow them to experience satisfaction and gain desired reinforcements by socially acceptable means (Henggeker et al., 1995).

4. *Community Centers.* Helping children develop appropriate social skills, such as working together; participating in decision making; making plans, discussing, and successfully completing plans (Wodarski & Wodarski, 1993).

5. *Outpatient Clinics and Treatment Facilities.* Helping clients reduce anxiety; eliminate disturbing behavioral problems; define goals in terms of career and lifestyle; increase self-esteem; gain employment; solve problems (both concrete and interpersonal); develop satisfying lifestyles; and learn skills necessary for successful adult functioning in society.

Adults. All technologies should be developed within a cognitive behavioral paradigm and operate within the basic theoretical frameworks that when cognitions change along with behaviors, then probability of behavioral change is increased, as is maintenance of the change.

1. *Family Service.* Helping in the development of marital interactional skills for effective problem solving and goal setting behaviors; development of better parenting behaviors; and development of better communication.

2. *Community Mental Health Centers.* Helping individuals reduce anxieties through relaxation techniques. Teaching self-control to enable clients to alter certain problem-causing behaviors. Offering assertiveness training as one means of having personal means met. Helping in the acquisition of behaviors to facilitate interaction with family, friends, and co-workers (Schulte et al., 1992; Wilson, 1996).

3. *Psychiatric Hospitals.* Using token economies to help clients acquire necessary prosocial behaviors for their effective reintegration into society. Structuring clients' environments through provision of reinforcement by significant others for the maintenance of appropriate social behaviors, such as self-care, employment, and social interactional skills. Analogous emphasis is indicated for working with persons classified as mentally retarded in institutions (Bond et al., 1995; Stein & Test, 1980).

4. *Public Welfare*. Helping clients achieve self-sufficiency; learn effective child management and financial management procedures; and develop social behaviors, skills and competencies needed to gain employment.
5. *Corrections, Halfway Houses and Treatment Centers*. Using token economies to increase prosocial behaviors; learn new job skills; and develop self-control and problem-solving strategies.
6 *Hospitals*. Using social learning theory for the treatment of cardiac disorders, chronic pain, headaches, diet disorders, obesity and smoking.

Implementation of Change Strategy: Level of Intervention

Social work has been characterized historically as a profession that emphasizes a one-to-one relationship with clients to achieve behavioral change (Glenn & Kunnes, 1973; Levine & Perkins, 1987; Ryan, 1971; Wodarski, 1997). However, the profession has seldom addressed itself adequately to the appropriateness of the various service-delivery mechanisms of certain types of clients. Few empirical studies have delineated the parameters or criteria for determining whether one-to-one group-level treatment is best for achieving behavioral changes in a given situation. Recent research indicates that the majority of intervention can be delivered in a group context with similar results (Fuhriman & Burlingame, 1994).

For example, training in relaxation, systematic desensitization, mindfulness-based cognitive therapy, self-esteem building, assertiveness, and parenting skills can all occur in one-to-one contexts. From a social learning theory perspective, however, it is posited that if a behavior is learned in a group context, it is likely to come under the control of a greater number of discriminative stimuli; therefore, greater generalizations of the behavior can occur for a broader variety of interactional contexts. There are additional substantiated rationales for working with individuals in groups. Groups provide a context where behaviors can be tested in a realistic atmosphere. Clients can get immediate peer feedback regarding their problem-solving behaviors. They are provided with role models to facilitate the acquisition of requisite social behavior. Groups provide a more valid focus for accurate diagnosis and a more potent means for changing client behavior (Baez, 2003; Fennell, 2004; Halla & Tarrier, 2002; Jones, 2001; Meyer & Smith, 1977; Rose, 1977; Westwood et al., 2003).

These theoretical rationales indicate that treating clients in groups should facilitate the acquisition of socially relevant behavior. In addition, group treatment is equally effective as individual service. Thus, managed care will support the use of groups to provide service. However, criteria need to be developed concerning who can benefit from group treatment. Such knowledge will only be forthcoming when adequately designed research projects are executed in which clients are assigned randomly to individual and group treatment to control for confounding factors, such as type of behavior, age, sex, income level, academic and social abilities.

Macrolevel Intervention. If, following an assessment, a change agent finds that a client is exhibiting appropriate behaviors for his social context but that a treatment organization or institution is not providing adequate reinforcers for appropriate behaviors, or that it is punishing appropriate behavior, the change agent must then decide to engage in organizational or institutional change. This may involve changing a social policy, changing bureaucratic means of dealing with people, or other strategies. To alter an organization, the worker will have to study its reinforcement contingencies and assess whether or not he or she has the power to change these structures so that the client can be helped.

Relapse Prevention

Generalization and Maintenance of Behavior Change. Interventions at the macrolevel are increasingly critical, since follow-up data collected five years later on antisocial children who participated in a year-long behavior modification program that produced extremely impressive behavioral changes in the children indicate that virtually none of the positive changes were maintained (McCombs et al., 1978). Possibly, maintenance could be improved when change is also directed at macrolevels.

Considerable study is needed to delineate those variables that facilitate the generalization and maintenance of behavior change. These may include substituting "naturally occurring" reinforcers, training relatives or other individuals in the client's environment, gradually removing or fading the contingencies, varying the conditions of training, using different schedules of reinforcement, and using delayed reinforcement and self-control procedures (Csiernick & Troller, 2002; Kazdin, 1975a; Kazdin, 1975b; Laws, 1999; Wodarski, 1980).

Such procedures will be employed in sophisticated and effective social service delivery systems. Home visits, which were once the focus of practice, may also be employed in the future. Positive features of home visits include providing the opportunity to assess family interactions more adequately, and increasing in the probability of involving significant others in the treatment process, the opportunity to delineate attitudinal differences and how they affect therapy, their ability to increase the worker's influence potential, and so forth (Allen & Tracy, 2004; Behrens & Ackerman, 1956; Chappel & Daniels, 1970; Freeman, 1967; Hollis, 1972; Mickle, 1963; Moynihan, 1974; Richmond, 1971).

Summary: Practice Recommendations

Based on the available data, the following generalizations may be made regarding managed care treatment components.

1. Human service should be time limited.
2. Services should involve substantial structure in terms of roles of worker and client.
3. Techniques that have an accumulative database should be utilized.
4. Appropriate intervention strategies should be used; for example, individual, group or societal.
5. Behaviors acquired in clients as a result of therapy must be maintained once therapy is conducted. Therefore, appropriate maintenance procedures must be considered.

Conclusion

Psychosocial treatment is a large domain that is continuing to be expanded and explored. There is a clear need for further extensive research and empirical validation for the techniques that have a proven record of accomplishment. There is also a need to investigate those methods that hold promise and a need to recognize and eliminate the ineffectual attempts.

It is a challenge to employ a psychosocial approach because of its frequent breadth and depth of treatment configuration. It embraces the client's life and world on more levels than a singular modality. This can be problematic, but not necessarily impossible, in the current managed care system.

There are many more methods and techniques that have just begun to be noticed and researched. There is an ambiguous territory to be traversed between being open minded to something that holds potential, despite its irregularity or unconventional bent, and falling into being undisciplined and imprudent in the less than judicious application of hopeful techniques based on anecdote or fond desires.

Within the broader field of social work, psychosocial treatment configurations could be a cornerstone for an intervention approach. It can evolve into the best balance of hard science and client centered holistic treatment based on the relationship of therapeutic alignment. This versatile, accessible, and effectively eclectic modality is dynamic in acknowledging all levels of being human.

6 Behavioral Health

Adolescent*

Adolescent Substance Abuse and Health Risk Behaviors

Introduction

Since 1993, adolescent substance abuse has been increasing in frequency with approximately 25 percent of adolescents at risk for substance abuse and related health risk behaviors (Brown, 1990). In a national sample of twelfth grade students, 81.7 percent reported using alcohol, 65 percent reported smoking cigarettes, 49.6 percent reported using marijuana, and 8.7 percent reported using cocaine at least once in their lifetime. (Johnston et al., 1995). Moreover, over $270 million was spent in 1992 for adolescent inpatient and outpatient treatment for substance abuse (Gans et al., 1995). However, these statistics may under represent high-risk youths who have dropped out of school (USPHS, 1991).

New data shows that high school students are drinking and smoking less than they were 15 years ago, according to a survey by the Center for Disease Control and Prevention. Fewer are having sex and carrying weapons, as well. Forty-three percent of high school students reported current alcohol use, compared with 51 percent in 1991. More than 14,000 high school students took the National Youth Risk Behavior Survey in 2005. While many risky behaviors have gone down, the survey found that a lot of high school students continue to engage in behaviors that place them at risk for the leading causes of mortality and morbidity (Pickoff-White, 2006).

Background

Substance abuse has been shown repeatedly to follow a progression from cigarettes and/or alcohol, to marijuana and ultimately other illicit drugs (Adler & Kandel, 1981; Andrews et al., 1991; Ellickson et al., 1992; Kandel, 1975; Merrill, 1999; Welte & Barnes, 1985). As substance abuse progresses, other health risk behaviors simultaneously increase. It is estimated that three million

---

*   Chapter written with the assistance of: Marisha Robinson and Carolyn Williams.

youths using substances are at a high risk for other risky behaviors (Falco, 1992; James et al., 1996; Kersting, 2005). The most common co-morbid health risk behaviors include unsafe sexual behaviors, delinquency, difficulties in school, and suicide (Barone et al., 1995; Escobedo et al., 1997; Fagan et al., 1990; Farrell et al., 1992; Kann et al., 1998; Rosenbaum & Kandel, 1990; Shrier et al., 1997). Some research has also started to include nutrition risks as well (Moberg & Piper, 1998; Riggs, & Cheng, 1988; Sarigiani et al., 1999).

For this chapter, one of the most common health risk behaviors and one of the under-represented health risk behaviors will be discussed. Therefore, unsafe sexual behaviors and nutrition will be the focuses of health risk behaviors here. Figure 6.1 shows a visual representation of substance abuse progression and the health risk behaviors that will be discussed.

Smoking, even social smoking, carries risks. The negative effects of tobacco use go well beyond health problems. Mental health disorders have been strongly associated with smoking, especially among adolescents and young adults. The Harvard College Alcohol Study determined that student tobacco users are 4.62 times more likely to smoke marijuana and 3.6 times more likely to engage in high-risk drinking than are nonsmokers (Rigotti, 2000). Smokers are more likely to use illicit drugs than high-risk drinkers (Forster & Wolfson, 1998; Wetter et al., 1998). Smoking causes more than 440,000 U.S. deaths per year, accounting for one out of every five deaths (CDC, 2004).

While poor nutrition is the least represented health risk behavior in the existent literature, it has been known to be effected by substance

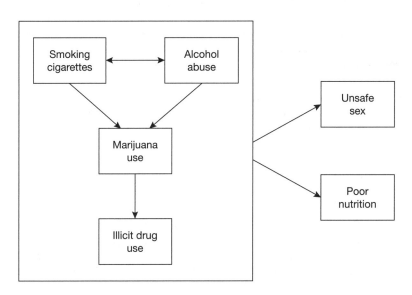

Figure 6.1 Conceptual Model of Adolescent Substance Abuse and Health Risk Behaviors

abuse behaviors (Watson & Mohs, 1989). For example, binge eating often accompanies marijuana use (Gross, et al., 1983; Hollister, 1971) and decreased nutritional intakes are often seen in illicit drug use where one may forget to eat, not feel hungry and/or use money to purchase drugs instead of healthy foods (Denny & Johnson, 1984).

The significance of understanding and researching health risk behaviors concurrent with substance abuse behavior is multifaceted. First, there is considerable evidence that initiation of substance abuse and health risk behaviors typically begins in adolescents, making this population the prime target for prevention (Warren et al., 1997). In addition, adolescents are further reinforced to engage in substance abuse use/health risk behaviors via social and peer acceptance, approval and popularity (Jessor, 1991). Second, research has shown that the earlier health risk behaviors begin, the more health problems an individual is likely to experience later in life (Dryfoos, 1990; 1991; Mott & Haurin, 1988). Examples of later life health troubles are cardio-vascular problems (Jessor, 1991). Finally, attempting to address behaviors that have not already been initiated is easier to accomplish than changing entrenched lifestyle behaviors (Warren et al., 1997). This has been shown in intervention research on sexual behaviors, smoking cigarettes and other substance abuse programs (Kirby et al., 1994; Orleans & Slade, 1993).

Smoking Prevalence

Approximately three million teens are smokers. It has been estimated that 10 percent of high school seniors smoke every day (Forster & Wolfson, 1998). These youths may preclude a variety of health problems, resulting in numerous economic problems for the individual, family, and society, by abstaining from smoking during adolescence.

Researchers link cigarette smoking in adolescence with excessive television viewing. The number of U.S. adolescents who smoke cigarettes has been increasing since 1991, with 70 percent of smokers becoming regular smokers by age 18. Youths who watch five or more hours of television per day are six times more likely to begin smoking than youths who watch less than two hours a day. Television, with its frequent portrayals of smoking as personally and socially rewarding, may be an effective indirect method of tobacco promotion, according to a recent study supported in part by the Agency for Health care Research and Quality (National Research Service Award training grant T32HS00063).

Roughly 88 percent of adult smokers began during adolescence, with most beginning at the ages of 11 and 15 (Bauman & Phongsavan, 1999; Yu & Williford, 1992). Seeing that many adult smokers began to use cigarettes in youth (Prince, 1995; Rigotti et al., 1997; Seffrin & Bailey, 1985) it is substantially cost-effective and productive to focus smoking prevention and cessation interventions in this age group. Elixhauser (1990) proposes that cessation of smoking during adolescence can negate 67 percent of lifetime smoking costs. Therefore, it is important for both youth and society to target youth with prevention and cessation programs.

Researchers led by Pradeep P. Gidwani, M.D., M.P.H. of Children's Hospital and Health Center in San Diego, CA used data from the National Longitudinal Survey of Youth, Child Cohort to examine the association of television viewing (based on an average of adolescent and parent reports) in 1990 among 592 youths aged 10 to 15 years with smoking initiation from 1990–1992. In 1990, one third of the youths watched more than five hours of television per day, and one tenth watched zero to two hours per day.

Among these young people overall, smoking increased from 4.8 percent in 1990 to 12.3 percent in 1992. Youths who watched more than 4 to 5 hours of TV per day were 5.2 times more likely to start smoking than those who watched television zero to two hours per day; young people who watched more than two to three hours were two times as likely. Television viewing may serve as a market for youths to exhibit high-risk behaviors such as smoking. Alternatively, television may substitute for activities that build resilience and help young people guard against high-risk behaviors.

The current findings concerning adolescent smoking state that peer smoking was by far the strongest predictor of smoking progression. Students that had at least two friends who smoked were more than six times as likely to transition from experimental smoking (do not smoke regularly) to intermittent smokers (smoking between one and 29 times out of the past 30 days).

Starting to smoke was more than nine times as likely among students drinking alcohol at least twice a month than it was among abstinent students. Furthermore, regular smoking was more than four times as likely among students drinking alcohol at least twice a month than it was among students who did not drink.

Adolescents from different minority groups (African American, Hispanic, and Asian) had decreased odds of transitioning to a higher smoking stage than White students. (But adult African Americans are more likely to smoke than Whites according to the Center for Disease Control.) But students who had a poor connection with school were more likely to try smoking and transition to become regular smokers, and those in the higher grades were also more likely to transition from smoking to regular/established smoking.

Smoking as a Gateway Drug

Smoking has been implicated as a gateway drug by several researchers. These findings have been sustained over time. In their study, Durant et al. (1999), found that youths who were smoking before or at age 11 were the most risk for future substance abuse, and health risk behaviors before age 15 are at the highest risk for subsequent risky behaviors and illicit drug use (Dishion & Andrews, 1995; Robins & Przybeck, 1985).

There are several contentions with the gateway theory, thus impacting the predictability of smoking as "The Gateway Drug." For example, some studies have shown alcohol to impact subsequent drug use and other risky health behaviors more than cigarettes (Kandel et al., 1992). Also, there are controversies about some youths who smoke, but who do not attempt to use other hard-core drugs (Merrill et al., 1999). These concerns are discussed in more detail in the theory section of this chapter.

Alcohol

Approximately 54 percent of eighth grade youth, 72 percent of eleventh grade youth and 82 percent of twelfth grade report having consumed alcohol at least once (Johnston et al., 1998). Making matters complicated, alcohol consumption has evolved into a developmental psychological behavior, or a right-of-passage, during adolescence and into early adulthood (Wodarski & Feit, 1995).

Studies have shown that persons who are chronic heavy drinkers are at great risk for changes in behavior and mental functioning (Kaplan & Sadock, 1991). This may cause increased risks to adolescents, many of whom are still developing physically, psychologically, and emotionally. As well, alcohol consumption in adolescence increases mental health problems, behavioral problems, school troubles, increased legal involvement, and actions that may prematurely affect the future. For example, neurotransmitters also indicated in mental health functioning, such as dopamine and serotonin, are affected by alcohol consumption (Carboni et al., 1989; Wozniak et al., 1990). Youths who are compromised cognitively, behaviorally, and psychologically are at more risk for exploring other risky health behaviors and may find themselves in life compromising situations.

Alcohol Abuse as a Gateway Drug

Research has shown that early alcohol use is known to be a precursor to illicit drug use and other health risky behaviors such as unsafe sex, delinquency, violent behaviors, and suicide (Brener & Collins, 1998; DuRant et al., 1997; DuRant et al., 1997b; Spingarn & DuRant, 1996; Woods et al., 1997). Much of this research is founded in gateway theory. As stated earlier, however, there is contention in the literature on alcohol or cigarettes being THE gateway drug. Some research addresses this by including both alcohol and cigarettes at the same influential point for subsequent drug use and other risky behaviors (Andrews et al., 1991; Ellickson et al., 1992). This is the supposition taken in this chapter as shown in Figure 6.1.

Marijuana

Marijuana use in adolescence typically occurs following the use of alcohol and/or cigarettes, according to gateway and problem behavior theory. There is substantial evidence that adolescents' use of marijuana is on the rise. For example, it has been noted in 1991 that 10 percent of eighth graders, 23 percent of tenth graders, and 37 percent of twelfth graders had tried using marijuana, while in 1997, 23 percent of eighth graders, 42 percent of tenth graders and 50 percent of twelfth graders admit to having tried using marijuana (Johnston, 1996; UMNIS, 1997). If one takes into account the gateway theory, then it is conceivable that many of these youths are also abusing/using alcohol and/or cigarettes.

It is commonly assumed that marijuana is non-addictive and non-health threatening by many adolescents (41.9%), however that is not the case (UMNIS, 1997). It is possible to become addicted to marijuana. Also there is evidence that continual use of the drug has similar health effects as smoking cigarettes and influences a decrease in immune system functioning (AAP, 1999; Cabral, 1996; Cottrell et al., 1973). Furthermore adolescent marijuana use may have other deleterious effects resulting from puberty such as impaired sperm production and ovulation problems (Asch et al., 1981; Cohen, 1985).

Research has shown that babies born to women who used marijuana during their pregnancies display altered responses to visual stimuli, increased tremulousness and a high-pitched cry, which may indicate neurological problems in development (Lester & Dreher, 1989). During infancy and preschool years, marijuana-exposed children have been observed to have more behavioral problems than unexposed children and poorer performance on tasks of visual perception, language comprehension, sustained attention, and memory (Fried, 1995). In school, these children are more likely to exhibit deficits in decision-making skills, memory, and the ability to remain attentive (Cornelius et al., 1995).

Major psychological effects of marijuana use are panic and high states. One fourth of all first time users develop panic reactions. Weil (1970) found that approximately 75 percent of negative reactions to marijuana use were accounted for by panic states. Furthermore, panic states secondary to marijuana use is more likely to occur when use takes place in environments where use are considered deviant.

Marijuana is the most prevalent illicit drug used by teens because it is easily accessible. In fact 90 percent of high school seniors stated that obtaining marijuana is virtually trouble-free, and nearly 40 percent of tenth graders reported smoking marijuana in 1999. Teens who use this drug are more likely to initiate the use of other drugs (e.g., cocaine, heroin, and meth) (McDowell & Futris, 2002).

In certain studies, weight gain and increases in daily caloric consumption was noted after 3–7 weeks of exposure to marijuana (Foltin et al., 1986; Greenberg et al., 1976). The following nutritional deficiencies and ensuing symptoms have been noted in individuals who smoke marijuana: changes in appetite, muscle weakness, increased tiredness, abnormal breathing patterns when physically active, bleeding gums, indigestion, tongue soreness, low levels of zinc (Mohs et al., 1990). In a study of male adolescent marijuana and alcohol users, many youths had a below average intake of fruit, vegetables and milk. It was also noted that these youths had higher intakes of "junk foods" (Farrow et al., 1987).

Marijuana and Subsequent Health Risks Behaviors

It has been proposed that adolescent marijuana users are most likely to be respected by peers who also use marijuana and shunned by those who do not (DuRant et al., 1999). This may further predispose these youths to other risky behaviors, reinforced by their peer group such as future illicit drug use (Levy & Pierce, 1990; NIDA, 1980). Using marijuana has also been linked to an increased propensity to engage in unsafe sex practices, accidents and injuries (Irwin, 1989; Irwin & Ryan, 1989; Kokotailo & Adger, 1991).

Illicit Drug Use

As we consider the number of youths using marijuana, gateway theory and problem behavior theory suggest that youths are subsequently at risk for using illicit drugs such as cocaine (powder, crack), heroin, and meth. Not surprisingly, then, it has been noted by some researchers that 25 percent of tenth and twelfth grade youths admit to having used illicit drugs at least once in a 30 day period and 54.3 percent of twelfth grade youths report having tried an illicit drug during their lifetime (UMNIS, 1997). Despite these data, however it must be noted that most of these youths do not become dependent on drugs (Newcomb, 1995). This may suggest more experimental behavior versus underlying thrill seeking or risk taking predisposition as suggested in problem behavior theory.

Nasal heroin use increased double fold in the preadolescent population between 1991 and 1997 (UMNIS, 1997). The common fears associated with heroin such as HIV and hepatitis have diminished since sniffing heroin has become popularized, thus increasing adolescent usage (Bruner & Fishman, 1998). Nonetheless these youths are still at risk for HIV and other STDs. Using the drug may impair abilities to engage in safe sex practices and discernment regarding their sex partner(s).

By age fourteen 14.35 percent of youths have engaged in some form of illicit (illegal) drug use. By the end of high school, more than 50 percent will have used at least one illicit drug. Teens that begin using illicit drugs before the age of fifteen are more likely to develop a lifelong dependence on illegal substances. A few of the common drugs used by youth are marijuana, ecstasy, heroin, and cocaine (McDowell & Futris, 2002).

Illicit Drug Use and Subsequent Health Risk Behaviors

A co-morbid relationship exists between illicit drug use and unsafe sex, predisposing these youths not only to health consequences from the drugs, but also to STDs, HIV, and unplanned pregnancy (Bruner & Fishman, 1998;

Jessor & Jessor, 1998; Kann, et al., 1996; Kokotailo, 1995). There is also a relationship between illicit drug use and their other risky behaviors such as delinquency, truancy, weapon carrying, suicide and homicide (Kokotailo, 1995; Simon et al., 1998). Furthermore, as nutrition status in adolescent risky behaviors begins to be included in this research, new problems start to arise. For example, youths who use cocaine show a decrease in food intake, increased nutrient imbalance, and increased consumption of fatty foods (Jonas et al., 1987).

Approximately 12.5 percent of girls between the ages of 15 and 19 become pregnant yearly (MCH, 1995). Attention to adolescent sexual behavior is largely due to the rise in youths being diagnosed with HIV, STDs and pregnancy.

These issues not only affect the adolescent's health and future, but also impact the economy (NCHS, 1992) through loss of labor, medical costs, and public assistance. In 1988, Americans were spending approximately $175,000 annually for teen abortions and approximately $1.24 billion to treat low-birth-weight babies from adolescent mothers (Gans et al., 1995).

It is estimated that 12 million individuals under the age of 25 are diagnosed with an STD yearly. Furthermore, it is estimated that 25 percent of teens will be diagnosed with an STD by the time of high school graduation. Although difficult to estimate, approximately 1 percent of youth account for all reported cases of AIDS and this represents one of the most rapidly growing AIDS-infected populations. It must be added that this number does not represent the number of youths who potentially have HIV, probably reflecting confidentiality and ethical concerns pertaining specifically to youth. As well, research on the co-morbidity of adolescent substance use and HIV/AIDS is scarce (Jainchill et al., 1999). However, AIDS has been one of the leading causes of adolescent mortality (Strunin & Hingson, 1992). Furthermore, there is evidence that the prevalence of adolescent sexual activity is increasing with the majority of youth not using protection (OTA, 1991).

Those theorists who subscribe to problem behavior theory suggest abusing behaviors and unsafe sexual behaviors have the same underlying causes. These underlying causes perpetuate the initiation of healthy risky behaviors and then reinforce the continuation of these behaviors due to resulting "highs" from thrill seeking (Barnes & Welte, 1986; Elliot et al., 1985). This is discussed in more detail in the theory section of this chapter.

Co-morbid Risky Health Behavior: Poor Nutrition

The adolescent population has unique nutritional needs as they are going through significant physical and psychological changes often very rapidly. In some research, youth nutritional intakes in general have been reported below what is necessary for healthy growth (Driskell et al., 1987; Story & VanZyl York, 1987). Furthermore, there is evidence that high-risk youth have lower healthy nutritional levels that put them at a disadvantage for diet-related problems (Story, 1984).

In adolescence, dietary recommendations and needs may fluctuate, depending on gender and growth spurts. For example, males incurring a growth spurt may consume 4,000 kcals/daily to maintain weight, while a female who has completed her growth spurt may consume fewer than 2,000 kcals/daily, similar to recommendations. Nutritional needs for adolescents, therefore, cannot be generalized other than it varies between each individual.

A study conducted by Basen-Engquist et al. (1996), suggests three clusters of adolescent health risky behaviors that include nutritional risks: low school grades; little to no participation in sport activities; and poor nutritional status by changing food, water and salt intakes (Mohs et al., 1990). Also, substance use impacts weight and metabolism that can impact the overall health and well being of the individual (Mohs et al., 1990).

Cigarettes

Nicotine has been shown to decrease sugar consumption during a 20-minute interval where the individual was permitted to smoke. However, when the individual was not allowed to smoke, increase in sugar consumption was noted (Grunberg, 1982). Not surprisingly, therefore, it is very common to see weight gain in those who are trying to quit smoking (Rabkin, 1984). Depletion of micro-nutrients in the body were shown in smokers, as well as a decrease in vitamin E in lung fluids and an increased need for Vitamin C in the diet (Alonso-Aperte & Varela-Moreiras, 2000). Light cigarettes have been marketed by the tobacco industry as being a healthier smoking choice, a safe alternative to cessation, and a first step toward quitting smoking altogether. Research, however, has failed to show a reduction in smoking-related health risks, an increase in rates of smoking cessation, a decrease in the amount of carbon monoxide or tar released, or a reduction of cardiovascular disease or lung cancer associated with light cigarette use, compared with regular cigarette use.

Nevertheless, more than one-half of adolescent smokers in the United States smoke light cigarettes. The purpose of this article is to explore adolescents' perception of the risks associated with smoking light cigarettes, as well as adolescents' attitudes and knowledge about the delivery of tar and nicotine, health risks, social effects, addiction potential, and ease of cessation with light cigarettes, compared with regular cigarettes (Kropp & Halpern-Felsher, 2004).

Design

Participants were 267 adolescents (mean age: 14.0 years). The participants felt that they would be less likely to get lung cancer, have a heart attack, die from a smoking-related disease, get a bad cough, have trouble breathing, and get wrinkles when smoking light cigarettes. Furthermore when participants were asked how long it would take to become addicted to the two cigarette types (light versus regular), they thought it would take significantly longer to become addicted to light versus regular cigarettes.

Adolescents also thought that their chances of being able to quit smoking were higher with light versus regular cigarettes; similarly, when participants were asked how easy it would be to quit smoking light cigarettes than regular cigarettes. Overall, adolescents hold misconceptions in both their personal risk estimates and their general attitudes about health risks, addictive properties, and ease of cessation associated with light cigarettes.

Furthermore, there is evidence that adolescents are not fully aware of the addictive nature of cigarettes and therefore think that they can experiment with smoking during adolescence without becoming addicted or experiencing any health consequences.

Alcohol

Those who consume alcohol show signs of increased susceptibility to infections and alterations in immune system functioning, malnutrition, and malabsorption (Watson, 1988; 1992). Furthermore, it is not uncommon to see weight gain in individuals who consume large amounts of alcohol due to the biochemical properties of the substance (Denny & Johnson, 1984). In effect, those who use alcohol tend to eat less, secondary to large amounts of caloric intake from the substance, often resulting in poor nutrition. At times, yearning for alcohol can surpass the natural desire to eat further complicating the body's access to necessary nutrients (Denny & Johnson, 1984).

Heavy alcohol consumers tend to show decreased levels of vitamin B (Hoyumpa & Schenker, 1982), thiamin, folic acid and abnormal metabolism of vitamin B (Alonso-Aperte & Varela-Moreiras, 2000). Adolescent drinkers may be at increased susceptibility to nutritional effects of alcohol due to dieting, poor food choices and increased risk of pre-existing nutrient deficiencies that are commonly seen in this age group (Alonso-Aperte & Varela-Moreiras, 2000). However, there has been little to no empirical research done in the adolescent population to substantiate this.

It is not uncommon to see hepatitis, cirrhosis, ulcers, stomach/pancreas/intestinal swelling and brain damage in those who are alcohol dependent and long-time users. However, most of this research has been done in the adult population. There is limited information of these complications in the adolescent population.

Cocaine

Cocaine abuse impacts an individual's nutrition by decreasing food intake, increasing nutrition imbalance, and increasing the consumption of fatty foods. Not surprisingly there is a higher rate of anorexia nervosa (in humans) and malnutrition (in mice) subsequent to decreased eating (Jonas et al., 1987; Lopez et al., 1991). Watson & Mohs (1989) reported a 32 percent co-morbidity of anorexia nervosa and bulimia in individuals using cocaine. There is also evidence of cocaine abusing individuals.

Cocaine has been a serious drug problem in America for almost a century. According to the National Institute on Drug Abuse, 5 percent of twelfth graders reported using cocaine in 2000 (McDowell & Furtis, 2002).

While there have been limited studies focusing on the nutritional effects of heroin use, slow insulin responses and low potassium levels have been supported which may influence secondary heroin related health complications such as impaired kidney functioning, impaired skeletal muscle, and delayed glucose metabolism (Giugliano, 1984; Reed & Ghodse, 1973; Watson & Mohs, 1990).

Summary

The significance of understanding and researching health risk behaviors concurrent with substance abuse behavior is multifaceted. There is consider-able evidence that the initiation of substance abuse and health risk behaviors begins in adolescence, making this population the prime target for prevention. The earlier health risk behaviors are initiated, the more health problems an individual is likely to experience later in life. There is considerable evidence of substance using behaviors causing immediate health problems for adoles-cents who are at a greater risk for STDs, HIV/AIDS, poor nutrition and injuries. Research has shown that it is easier to prevent behaviors that have not already been initiated than to attempt to address lifestyle behaviors (Warren et al., 1997). This has been shown in intervention research on sexual behaviors, smoking cigarettes and other substance abuse programs (Kirby et al., 1994; Orleans & Slade, 1993). By teaching youths how to effectively avoid and refuse to engage in risky behaviors, we will avoid the medical, societal, psychological, and economic impact that these behaviors currently possess, thus promoting healthier and more productive young adults in the future.

Theoretical Models for Adolescent Health Risk Behaviors

Introduction

Three main adolescent health risk behavior theories presented in empirical literature will be defined and discussed. These include gateway theory, problem behavior theory and social influence theory. Criticisms of each theory are also presented.

A theoretical model is supposed to assist the researcher in understanding the etiology of a behavior and predicting the occurrence of that behavior. In this section, we will examine the major theories or models proposed to help us understand health risk behaviors in the adolescent population. Health risk behaviors include substance abuse, delinquency, unsafe sex, suicide, truancy, behavior problems, psychological problems, and poor nutritional habits. Several theories have proposed that these behaviors are related and predict the likelihood of adolescents engaging in more severe health risk behaviors. For example, an adolescent is more likely to use marijuana if they already are using or have experimented with cigarettes and/or alcohol. Three main theories have traditionally been used in health risk behavior research: gateway theory, problem behavior theory, and social influence theory. These three theories will be delineated and critically examined below.

Gateway Theory

Many studies have shown a sequential pattern in drug use that remained consistent over time and across populations, thus posting a focal point for prevention (Fisher et al., 1991; Merrill et al., 1999; Yamaguchki & Kandel, 1984). That is, initial use of alcohol or cigarettes leading to marijuana use and then progressing to more illicit drugs such as cocaine or heroin. Typically, concurrent increases in alcohol consumption and/or cigarette use is also seen as the individual starts to use other drugs (Adler & Kandel, 1981; Andrews et al., 1991; Ellickson et al., 1992; Kandel, 1975; Merrill et al., 1999; Welte & Barnes, 1985). Longitudinal and cross-sectional research that supports this progression has been conducted on gateway theory (Kandel & Davies, 1991; Kandel et al., 1992; Kandel & Yamaguchi, 1993; Yamaguchi & Kandel, 1984). Some researchers have noted that gateway theory is inclusive of risky behaviors that coincide with drug progression such as unsafe sex and delinquency (Fagan et al., 1990; Farrell et al., 1992; Rosenbaum & Kandel, 1990).

While gateway theory supports this pattern, it does not assume that all youths who smoke cigarettes or drink alcohol will progress to using drugs. It merely places these youths at higher risk for other drug use and risky behaviors, suggesting that other demographics are in play such as gender, socio-economic status, family dynamics and early behavior difficulties (Merrill et al., 1999; USGAO, 1993). For example, females appear to be more influenced for future drug use by smoking initiation rather than by alcohol. However, for males, alcohol appears to be the precursor for other drug involvement, with or without cigarette use (Kandel et al., 1992). Furthermore, some data suggests that the earlier alcohol and/or cigarette use is initiated, the more predisposed the youth is for illicit drug use and subsequent risky behaviors (Kandel et al., 1993; Merrill et al., 1999; Yu & Williford, 1994).

Those who criticize gateway theory point to limited empirical research resulting in insufficient data to infer a causal relationship for drug and risky behaviors (Merrill et al., 1999). Much of the existent research depends on cross-sectional data and therefore, causal conclusions cannot be made. However, there are some longitudinal studies that allow for more causal conclusions to be drawn. For instance, in their four-year research of gateway theory, Ellickson et al. (1992) were able to support the use of alcohol and cigarettes before the use of marijuana, followed by other illicit drug use over time. Their study also supported an increase in the use of non-illegal substances prior to illegal drug initiation.

Empirical gateway theory research is also limited in drug sequence differences based on ethnic background. For example, it is proposed that different ethnic backgrounds may be exposed to varying levels of specific kinds of drug use, increasing the probability of ethnic-specific drug sequences (Ellickson et al., 1992). However, Ellickson et al. (1992) noted similar drug sequence among adolescent Caucasian, African American, and Hispanics. The only exception to this was adolescent Asian Americans who typically used other substances first and alcohol last. Nonetheless, more research needs to be conducted in this area.

Another problem with gateway theory is predictive ability. Statistically, it has been shown that 44 percent of eighth grade youths have tried alcohol and 20 percent of eighth graders have been drunk at least once (Johnston et al., 2005). However, not all of these youths go on to use marijuana or other illicit drugs (Ellickson et al., 1992). Furthermore, those who appear to be most at risk for engaging in substance abusing behaviors may not do so due to resiliency, whereas others who do not appear to be at high risk may initiate substance abusing behaviors (Garmezy, 1991; Luthar & Ziegler, 1991; Resnick et al., 1997; Rutter, 1993). In attempts to address this problem, certain researches have been operationally defining behaviors. One study found that a tenth grade youth consuming an average of two alcoholic beverages weekly was more likely to progress to other drug abuse, and weekly cigarette smoking increased the likelihood of illicit drug use (Ellickson et al., 1992). The progression does not always follow the same pattern. Rather, the progression tends to follow the popularity of certain drugs at the time (Chaiken, 1993; Golub & Johnson, 1996, 1997; Hamid, 1992). However, the majority of this research has been limited to the increase of cocaine use.

While the gateway theory has enjoyed popular acceptance for some time, scientists have always had their doubts, and recently, these doubts were proven justified. After analyzing data from the United States National Household Survey on Drug Abuse, researchers found that teenagers who tried hard drugs were predisposed to do so whether or not they tried marijuana (www.norml.org, 2005). This conclusion produces doubts regarding the legitimacy of federal drug policies based upon the premise of this theory.

Problem Behavior Theory

One perspective that has been suggested in place of gateway theory is problem behavior theory. This theory proposes that certain youths are predisposed to drink and smoke. The same underlying dynamic also puts these youths at higher risk to engage in other hazardous behaviors (Donovan and Jessor,

1985; Donovan et al., 1988; Durant et al., 1999; Jessor, 1987, 1991). For example, there are studies indicating the co-morbidity of unsafe sex, substance abuse, poor nutrition, difficulties in school and criminal behavior among adolescents (Barone et al., 1995; Escobedo et al., 1997; Farrell et al., 1992; Kann et al., 1998; Shrier et al., 1997). Health beliefs of the adolescent are also tied into problem behavior theory as it is proposed that deviant/risky behaviors are more likely to occur when the individual does not place importance on their health (Wood et al., 1995).

The earlier risky behaviors are started, the more likely the individual is to engage in clusters of risky behaviors later (Durant et al., 1999; Jessor et al., 1991; Jessor, 1992). At-risk youths are disproportionately exposed to social environments where risky behaviors are expected and supported. The normative developmental adolescent process of separating from parents or individualizing reinforces this, a common underlying dynamic shared by risk behaviors (Jessor et al., 1991; Jessor, 1992). Some research has been able to support this supposition by presenting correlations between specified health risk behaviors (Basen-Engquist et al., 1996).

It has also been suggested that there are five factors that underlie the link between risky behaviors. These are: biology/genetics; how one views their environment; personality characteristics; living environment; and behavior. Some psychological risk factors have also been implicated including: expected results of engaging in the behavior; attitude; beliefs; values; and knowledge (Robinson et al., 1987).

One weakness in problem behavior research is limited data with different ethnic groups. In attempts to address this weakness, Mitchell and Beals (1997) conducted the first health risk behaviors study based on problem behavior theory with Native American adolescents. Results showed support for a clustering of risky behaviors in this population. Still, this was a preliminary study so more research needs to be conducted with inclusive focus on ethnic groups.

Another criticism of the theory is limited research and analysis to support the construct validity of risky behavior clusters (Mitchell & Beals, 1997). There have been some attempts to operationalize risky behaviors as antisocial, cannabis use, frequency of alcohol consumption, and engaging in sex (Donovan et al., 1988). While this is a start, definitional attempts fall short of being able to support construct validity. Due to the lack of ethnic group research under the assumptions of problem behavior theory, construct validity is further compromised. Future research attempts at strengthening the validity of the theory are needed.

One of the least studied health risk behaviors in adolescents is nutritional habits. The Youth Risk Behavior Surveillance studies incorporate nutritional risks (Everett et al., 1997; Grunbaum et al., 2000; Kann et al., 1993; Kann et al., 1998; Kolbe et al., 1993). However, these studies do not discuss a theoretical foundation. In a study by Nemark-Szainter et al. (1996), they did address unhealthy weight loss, but this is considered a more specified nutritional concern, not a global nutritional behavior.

Furthermore, the longevity of problem behavior theory is unclear. Most of the research has surrounded those between ages 12 and 18 and there is some question of how applicable this theory is into and throughout adulthood (McGee & Newcomb, 1992; Newcomb & Bentler, 1988). This is most often seen in longitudinal prevention programs where positive results during younger years are no longer seen in late adolescence/early adulthood. However, the literature is conflicted in this regard with Donovan et al. (1988), which finds problem behavior theory relevant into adulthood. There is also some evidence that younger youth may not be appropriately addressed by problem behavior theory.

There are other underlying causes for risky behaviors (Gillmore et al., 1991). McGee and Newcomb (1992) attempt to address developmental and underlying etiological questions in their study. They found that delinquency and sexual behaviors appear to be more influenced by different developmental age-frames. The developmental application of problem behavior theory to all age groups remains speculative.

There are emerging questions about the generalizability of problem behavior theory. It has been proposed that some risky behaviors may cluster around each other, but they are non-inclusive of all risky behaviors (McGee & Newcomb, 1992). For instance, there is great evidence that substance use correlates with risky sexual behavior, delinquency and poor academic goals (Donovan & Jessor, 1985; Jessor & Jessor, 1977; Newcomb & Bentler, 1986; Newcomb et al., 1989). But, these clusters of risky behaviors may not be correlated with other clusters such as substance use and poor nutritional habits.

Despite their differences, gateway theory and problem behavior theory can be compatible as they both attempt to understand the etiology of risky health behaviors. Having a sound comprehension of adolescent substance abuse initiation allows for a better foundation for preventive program development (Graham et al., 1991a).

Social Influence Theory

Gateway theory and problem behavior theory introduce intriguing and relevant concepts toward better etiological and foundational understanding of substance abuse progression and concurrent health risk behaviors. However, these theories are limited in their contributions toward implementing effective preventive interventions because they mainly try to answer the question, "What are the factors that allow the progression of substance abuse?" (Kim et al., 1998). For this reason, a great deal of adolescent behavior prevention literature also incorporates a social influence model. Social influence is "the modern, scientific study of persuasion, compliance, propaganda, 'brainwashing', and the ethics that surround these issues" (www.workingpsychology.com, 2002).

In 1981, Latané conceptualized several main components of social impact; these include helping, crowding, social inhibition and social pressure conformity (Witte, 1990). Future research then identified social impact, social inhibition, social loafing and social facilitation as other factors to consider in social impact theory (Witte, 1990). As researchers began to criticize social impact theory, the social influence model (Tanford & Penrod, 1984) and group situation theory (Witte, 1987) emerged. Three main components of social influence theory that impact adolescent substance use have been defined by Graham et al. (1991b): (1) offers to try a substance; (2) modeling of substance using behaviors; and (3) misconstrued understanding of actual peer substance use.

The premise of the social influence model is that youths start to use substances as a result of positive messages they hear about drugs and alcohol from family, adults, peers and the media. Based on these findings, program development researchers have incorporated resistive skills, education, peer competitions, teaching youths how to analyze the media and advertising, and encouraging community support/involvement (Beane, 1990; Moberg & Piper, 1998; Slavin et al., 1990; Stephenson, 1991; Howard, 1992). At times, the social influence model is utilized conjunctive to cognitive-behavioral models. This combination has been shown to be effective with unsafe behavior prevention efforts (Schinke, 1982).

One major precept in this model is avoiding substance use and other risky behaviors through positive modeling and positive reinforcement from peers in social situations (Botvin et al., 1995; Evans et al., 1978). In their study, Donaldson et al. (1994) reported that the social influence model appears to encourage social norms that discourage adolescent substance use initiation. The results are a decrease in youth intrigue as the behavior is viewed as socially unacceptable.

At times, social influence theory can be too broad in definition. For example, it has been noted by some researchers that social influence can include all areas of social psychology (Worchel et al., 1988). Taking this into consideration, the operational definition or parameters of social influence theory within social psychology is difficult to ascertain (Levy, 1998). It may be that more specific definitions of the theory are generated by the applicability to precise topic areas. However, this brings up the question, "Is social influence a theory?"

Social influence theory does not indicate when and where certain aspects or definitive characteristics need to be included (Levy et al., 1998). Yet, most theorists will agree on specific qualifying criteria to define social influence. Some researchers have indicated two different subgroups under the term social influence theory. These include compliance-identification-internalization trichotomy (Kelman, 1958, 1961) and six power bases: coercive; reward; legitimate; referent; expert; and informational (French, 1956; French & Raven, 1959; Raven 1965). These subgroups were studied and defined about 40 years ago. Current social influence theory researchers need to address these concerns, especially if the theory is being highly used as a foundation for intervention creation. In their research, Levy et al. (1998) attempted to update the subgroups and to operationally define core elements of social influence theory. Their work has specified the following in relation to social influence theory: (1) cognitive processing ability and (2) how the individual perceives the intention of those influencing them and "direction of change" (the individual may react adversely or positively to the influencing stimuli). These specified parameters of social influence theory appear to be most applicable to adolescent substance abuse and health risk behavior prevention interventions.

Summary

Gateway and problem behavior theories have made a great impact in the etiological understandings of the progression of risky health behavior. However, the gateway theory has since been disproved and the problem behavior theory needs to be further substantiated through designs and analyses that allow causal interpretations to be drawn. Following etiological understanding, social influence theory attempts to create a sound foundation in preventative program development for adolescents. Programs based on social influence have been the most effective in the literature; however, more current research is needed to address an operationalized definition of social influence theory that can apply to interventive studies.

Preventing Adolescent Risky Behaviors

Introduction

Prevention research in risky health behaviors in adolescents began to take precedence in the 1970s. Each behavior has a different prevention history. The historical background of prevention programs for substance use, sexual behavior and nutrition habits will be discussed in the following section. After that, prevention programs in general will be critically discussed.

Historical Background

Tobacco

In 1970, television smoking ads were forbidden as a result of the Public Health Cigarette Smoking Act of 1969. The tobacco industry has vehemently disclaimed targeting teens; however, advertisements have been oriented toward youth (Forster & Wolfson, 1998; Stimmel, 1996). Recently, major cigarette companies have admitted to advertising to youth. They have also legally agreed to stop all advertising geared toward youth. In time, we will see how this impacts the proportion of teenage smokers.

In a study on mass media's effectiveness in decreasing cigarette smoking in adults and children, researchers found focus on second-hand smoke to be the most efficacious approach. They found that the teens in their study initiated smoking as a means of showing autonomy and rebelling against their parents. Mass media directed at teens was most effective in decreasing cigarette smoking when showing how the tobacco companies use advertising to coerce adolescents to smoke because the teens were able to see that they are not showing autonomy in smoking behavior if the tobacco companies are coercive (Forster & Wolfson, 1998).

In 1964, the Surgeon General called for anti-smoking campaigns in order to initiate cessation program attempts and decrease the health risks from smoking. By 1997, the Food and Drug Administration made it illegal for sellers of tobacco products to vend to teens under the age of 18 (Rigotti et al., 1997). Despite efforts, many sellers of tobacco products continue to sell to underage teens. In their study, Rigotti et al. (1997) found that regardless of improved compliance to the laws restricting sales to underage teens, adolescents did not report a decrease in cigarette purchases. More current findings suggest that variations in cigarette access may contribute differences in pupil smoking rates within schools, and that the relationship between access and adolescent smoking is circular, with greater availability increasing rates, and higher rates enhancing access (Turner et al., 2004).

Research shows evidence that youth smoking interventions backed by policies are the most productive (U.S. Department of Health and Human Services, 1997). An example of this is the formation of the Agency for Health Care Policy and Research, created by federal government legislation (Wetter et al., 1998). Focus on smoking cessation by this agency began in 1994. This resulted in the "Smoking Cessation Clinical Practiced Guideline" which provides scientifically based recommendations for conducting smoking cessation interventions (Wetter et al., 1998). One difficulty in making interventions accessible, however, is that most managed care companies put a damper on preventative services that are offered.

Some policies have been initiated on the federal level such as the Reorganization Act or Synar Amendment (Forster & Wolfson, 1998). The Reorganization Act "requires states to adopt laws prohibiting the sale and distribution of tobacco products to minors under 18, to implement central and local enforcement programs, and to provide annual reports to the DHHS demonstrating compliance." Another aspect of the Act mandates states to provide data regarding the decrease in cigarette smoking in teens throughout a four-year duration. Part of the Synar Amendment makes it possible for the federal government to impose punitive measures on anyone selling cigarettes to teens. If states do not provide evidence of attempts to reduce adolescent access to cigarettes via sales, then punitive measures, such as no access to block-grant funding, may be enforced (Rigotti et al., 1997).

Alcohol Prevention

In the 1970s, alcohol prevention studies were largely initiated as well as national tracking surveys to follow alcohol consumption by adolescents (Johnston et al., 1995). For the most part, these programs started out in schools and continue to prefer that milieu (Seffrin & Bailey, 1985; Wodarski & Feit, 1995). In the 1980s, parents and/or families were included in adolescent alcohol prevention programs (USDHHS, 1997).

There is contention in the literature about school-based prevention program effectiveness. For example, the popularized DARE program has been shown by some research to be non-effective in preventing substance abuse. However, a positive example is Teams-Games-Tournaments (TGT) which has been shown to be a powerful intervention to address teenage drinking (Wodarski & Feit, 1995; Wodarski, 1990; Wodarski, 1992–1993). This is a behavioral modification-based program which utilizes peer assistance with "group rewards" (Wodarski & Feit, 1995; Wodarski, 1988).

> TGT was developed through extensive research on games as teaching devices using small groups as classroom work units and emphasizing the task-and-reward structures used in the traditional classroom. The TGT technique is an alternative teaching approach that fully utilizes structure emphasizing group, rather than individual, achievement.
>
> (Wodarski, 1988, p. 48)

This technique has proved successful in adolescent drinking (Wodarski, 1988) and may be applicable with other adolescent addictive behaviors such as smoking cessation.

Illicit Drug Use Prevention

In 1937, the Marijuana Tax Act was enacted to deter individuals from growing, selling and using marijuana. One of the instigating factors leading to this legislation was the belief by Harry Anslinger, America's Commissioner of the Federal Bureau of Narcotics, that marijuana would be damaging to America's adolescent population (Rosenbaum, 1998). The Act had effectively dissuaded youth from engaging in marijuana use until the drug became popularized in the 1960s. Since then, presidential administrations have made "the war on drugs" a primary concern. Consequently, we have seen the initiation and continual evolution of adolescent substance abuse prevention programs that focus on cigarettes, alcohol, marijuana, LSD, heroin and amphetamines (Rosenbaum, 1996). In 1986, the U.S. reported spending $1.6 billion on substance abuse prevention and treatment (ADAMHA, 1991). Approximately $2.4 billion are spent yearly on substance prevention program for adolescents alone (U.S. General Accounting Office, 1997). Although several prevention programs have been cut, the government still offers many grants, particularly to school systems. Programs authorized under the Title IV, Safe and Drug-Free Schools and Communities Act (under the Elementary and Secondary Education Act of 1965) provide financial assistance for state and local drug and violence prevention activities in elementary and secondary schools, and institutions of higher education (U.S. Department of Education, 2005).

Risky Sexual Behavior Programs

Since 1981, the U.S. Office of Adolescent Pregnancy Programs (OAPP), through Title XX of the Public Health Services Act, has offered funding for research devoted to the development of sexual programs for adolescents (Jorgensen, 1991). Largely, OAPP funding has been limited to abstinence promotion versus safe sex education that includes information on contraception, planned pregnancy, abortion and sexually transmitted diseases, including HIV. This is because many parents are concerned about how much sexual information their children are exposed to. However, in this literature review, approximately half the articles found were focused on pregnancy prevention via contraception.

Many sex-prevention programs are educationally based; however, some critics indicate that this may not be the best approach. Not only has most past empirical research on sexual abstinence been shown to have questionable results (Hofferth & Miller, 1989), it has also been noted that many sexual abstinence programs, disseminated educationally and relying on cognitive processes, are unable to show significance due to the adolescent's inability to foresee consequences of behavior choices (Howard & McCabe, 1992). At times, the social influence model is utilized conjunctive to cognitive-behavioral models. This combination has been shown to be effective with unsafe sex behavior prevention (Schinke, 1982).

During the past five years, research has taken a more integrative approach. Pregnancy prevention programs largely focus on educating youths about contraceptive use, strategies for saying "no" to unsafe sex practices, including an abstinence component, and education about how pregnancy typically impacts the future (i.e. employment, income, education). Safe sex education and sexual abstinence promotion are being combined and integrated into most school systems. This is due, in large part, to adolescent abstinence research during the late 1970s and 1980s. Since then, researchers have been attempting to improve abstinence programs, as most studies prior to the 1990s have been non-effective or inconclusive. Furthermore, replication research has shown similar results, indicating less probability that non-effective or inconclusive study results were due to Type I error, methodological inconsistency or other factors (Wodarski & Wodarski, 1995).

Nutritional Programs

In the 1970s and 1980s, national nutritional surveys revealed that adolescents were not consuming adequate amounts of necessary foods for proper growth (Carroll et al., 1983; Fulgoni & Mackey, 1991). In the 1980s, the Comprehensive School Health Education Program was implemented in the school system (Harris, 1988). This program is structured to include youth from kindergarten through twelfth grade and contains the following components: community health, environmental health, development and growth, family life, consumer health, personal health, nutrition in the school and food service, disease control and prevention, prevention of accidents, promotion of safety and substance use/abuse (Allensworth & Kolbe, 1987; Frank 1998).

Despite the inclusion of substance use/abuse and nutrition in the school health education program, there is a gap in the empirical literature; these two behaviors were not integrated in prevention programs. Future prevention research needs to include nutrition habits of youth as a risk behavior. Proper nutrition has been shown to maintain good health and to decrease the likelihood of later life-altering/life-threatening illnesses, such as cardiovascular problems (Frank, 1998). Experimentation with substances and/or engaging in other health risk behaviors, such as unsafe sex, compounds this.

Discussion of Prevention Programs

It has been theorized that there are underlying motivations for youth to engage in risky behaviors and prevention programs for these behaviors tend to incorporate numerous sources of support. For example, it is not uncommon to see health risk behavior prevention programs that utilize school, peer, community, physician, family or any combination thereof as part of the intervention (Hawkins et al., 1999). Most often, however, interventions take place in a school setting (Donaldson et al., 1994).

From an epidemiological perspective on health risk behavior development in adolescents, behavioral and social influences are often cited as the most significant predictors (Jessor, 1991). Much literature suggests that the most predominant risk factors are influences from peers who are already using substances (Brook et al., 1990; Newcomb & Bentler, 1986). It appears, however, that coupling family and school interventions yields the most positive results (Resnick et al., 1997).

Since the 1970s, the majority of prevention research has focused on the etiology of adolescent substance abuse and related health risk behaviors. Prevention research has evolved from the gateway theory to problem behavior theory and, finally, to a public health prevention model that pays particular attention to risk factors and protective factors in youth regarding health risk behavior (Farquhar et al., 1990; Hawkins et al., 1999). A social influences model often accompanies these theories as a foundation for the intervention (Ary et al., 1990; Botvin et al., 1995; Ellickson et al., 1993; Hansen, 1992; Moberg & Piper, 1998; Hawkins et al., 1999; Schinke et al., 1988).

There is limited integration of etiological theories for health risk behaviors and the theories typically utilized in prevention programs. Many articles will mention the etiological theories in the introduction, but do not attempt to address the jump from those theories to the theoretical foundation of their program development. One exception to this is Life Skills Training techniques that have a strong foundation in problem behavior theory and are subsequently applied as prevention efforts (Botvin, 1985; Botvin, Baker et al., 1984a; 1984b).

It has only been with the inclusion of social influence theory that research has focused on techniques geared toward decreasing or eliminating adolescent substance abuse and concurrent health risk behaviors. In other words, earlier research was more explorative in nature and based on risk factors, whereas state-of-the-art research is more substantial and based on promoting youth empowerment (Kim et al., 1998).

In the social influence model, the implications of health behavior decisions are of primary focus for teens. Seldom do youth between the ages of 11 and 14 make health decisions based on health beliefs or information, but rather on social settings and peer groups surrounding them when the decision is made (Brown, 1990; Millstein & Litt, 1990; Moberg & Piper, 1998). The social influence model suggests that school support against health risk behaviors often strengthens youth ability to withstand pressures to engage in them (Resnick et al., 1997).

For the most part, prevention studies have been based on cognitive learning and provide sixth and seventh grade youths with facts in an attempt to increase awareness and prevention of health risk behaviors (Eisen et al., 1990; Grimley & Lee, 1997; Olsen et al., 1992). However, the literature has shown that youths do not typically respond well to this type of intervention longitudinally and showed marginal results during immediate follow-up analysis (Bell et al., 1993; Bruvold, 1993; Klitzner et al., 1991; Resikow & Botvin, 1993; Tobler, 1992).

When social influence theory is integrated into program development, 63 percent of programs showed positive results, 26 percent showed neutral results and 11 percent showed negative results (Hansen, 1992). While these results are far from being ideal, they are more efficacious than those programs based on education alone (Eisen et al., 1990; Olsen et al., 1992; Roosa & Christopher, 1990). It has been further proposed that insufficient analysis on possible spurious relationships may influence the frequency of intervention failure (McCaul & Glasgow, 1985). Further research investigating other interceding factors may help to improve the effectiveness of prevention programs.

Research utilizing more active approaches such as groups, peer competitions and focusing on skill development have shown more promising results in changing health risk behavior with adolescents (Barry, 2006; Moberg & Piper, 1998). Furthermore, eight instructing methods have been identified in the literature as the most effective for health behaviors with teenagers. These include peer leaders, parent interviews, social and refusal skills, health promotion, focusing on immediate effects of choosing certain health behaviors, feedback regarding peer norms, public commitments and teaching youths how to analyze the media and advertising (Beane, 1990; Howard, 1992; Moberg & Piper, 1998; Slavin et al., 1990; Stephenson, 1991).

Despite overwhelming literature showing the pattern of drug use and subsequent health risk behaviors, very limited research has been conducted toward preventing health risk behaviors as a whole. There is, however, research pointed at the prevention of specific health risk behaviors. For example, there are studies that focus particularly on adolescent substance abuse prevention and STD/HIV prevention, but few studies that attempt to address clusters of health risk behaviors found in etiological research. For example, Basen-Engquist et al. (1996) suggest three clusters of adolescent health risk behaviors that include nutritional risks: (1) low school grades, little to no participation in sport activities and poor nutritional habits as evidenced by limited fruit and vegetable intake; (2) limited exercise and high-fatty diet; and (3) dieting habits that are health threatening, smokeless tobacco use, motorcycle riding without a helmet and swimming without supervision. Furthermore, there are numerous studies based on gateway theory that mainly address the prevention of smoking cigarettes, but few that integrate problem behavior theory by addressing concurrent substance abuse and health risk behaviors longitudinally (Bell et al., 1993; Moberg & Piper, 1998; Shope et al., 1998).

In an attempt to be as comprehensive as possible in preventing substance abuse and other health risk behaviors in adolescents, including nutritional needs, the American Medical Association has developed the Guidelines for Adolescents Preventive Services (GAPS) program (AMA, 1996, 1997). This intervention is structured to promote avoidance of health risk behaviors, to increase awareness of existing behavioral, emotional or physical problems, to ensure youths are properly immunized and to promote the maintenance of healthy behaviors (Levenberg & Elster, 1995a, 1995b; Marquis & Wagner, 1997).

One shortcoming of the above-mentioned approaches to prevention is that they do not consider the nature of American society. It has been proposed that America is a drug culture, as many adults use caffeine, alcohol, cigarettes, and prescribed medications. For adolescents, this may confuse the distinction between legal and illicit drugs (Rosenbaum, 1998). Furthermore, it may be assumed, due to adolescent cognitive development, that youths have more difficulty distinguishing appropriate usage and misuse of legal drugs.

Adolescence is typically a time for experimentation, so defining substance abuse as deviant behavior may be another shortcoming. Youths living within a society that frequently uses substances may experiment with substances as a normal developmental process (Shedler & Block, 1990). It may be that we do not see higher success rates of prevention programs because these concerns are often neglected. To this degree, it has been proposed that prevention programs focus on harm reduction instead of abstinence (Rosenbaum, 1998).

Summary

While most adolescent prevention studies were initiated in the late 1970s, we are just beginning to see more positive results than negative results. However, these programs continue to show more success immediately after exposure to the intervention and do not seem to be maintained long-term. Future research needs to incorporate the natural development and progression of substance use, nutritional habits and sexual behavior within the context of American society into the assessment of success in prevention programs. Furthermore, there is limited integration of nutritional needs, education and unhealthy eating prevention in health risk behavior programs. Future research needs to address this area, as nutrition has been shown to prevent other life-threatening illnesses later in life and may be part of overall health risk behavior clusters.

7 Adult Behavioral Health*

No single theory dominates research or practice (Glantz et al., 1990). Theories explain or predict future actions. Theories tell us about the what, how, when, and why and help in the selection of appropriate interventions and the implementation of educational programs (Glantz et al., 1990). This section will outline a variety of theories that are applicable to behavioral medicine such as: Behavioral Medicine Paradigm, Theory of Reasoned Action, Multi-attribute Utility Theory, Attribution Theory, Consumer Information Processing, Social Learning Theory, and Trans-theoretical Model.

Behavioral Medicine Paradigm

Pinkerton et al. (1982) refer to behavioral medicine as the clinical application of principal techniques and procedures of social learning theory in the assessment, treatment management, rehabilitation, and prevention of disease (DeAngelis, 2005). This includes the behavioral reactions to physical dysfunction. The validations of such treatment techniques are researched through systematic investigations.

Assumptions

1 Physical problems are often related to lifestyle and individual's interactions with the environment (Raines & Erickson, 1997).
2 Depends upon careful analysis of all of the factors in relation to disease etiology and maintenance of health (Pinkerton et al., 1982).
3 Replaces the single cause models of disease, such as germ models of causation, with a multifaceted etiological model (McClelland, 1989).
4 In order to be successful, new disciplinary fields are forming, breaking the traditional boundaries between disciplines (Wodarski et al., 1991;

* Chapter written with the assistance of: Shawn Lawrence, Kim Zittel-Palamara, Beth Catchot, Matthew Hunt, and Nikki Walles.

Wodarski, 2000). These disciplines include psychobiology, sociobiology, and behavioral medicine.

5   The most important factor in developing a behavioral modification therapy strategy is a complete and individualized assessment of the behavior that is to be changed. The assessment specifies the target problem and indicates the conditions that constitute a resolution of the problem (Wodarski et al., 1991). Pinkerton and colleagues (1982) suggest four steps to a comprehensive behavioral assessment: define, specify antecedents, quantify target behaviors, and specify desired outcomes.

6   Self-monitoring is frequently used in the assessment of behaviors. This involves the client's observations and recordings of behavior antecedents and consequences. This brings the antecedents and consequences into the individual's awareness (Blanchard & Schwartz, 1988; Prochaska, 1998). Though this method does bring antecedents and consequences to the client's awareness, self-report is not always accurate and often can facilitate change in it.

7   Cognitive variables meditate behavior. Consequently cognitive strategies are now integrated with most behavioral medicine strategies. Principles showing that learning may occur through the observation of others (modeling) is also incorporated into this theory (Bandura, 1977).

Critique

Taking this theory into account, both the individual and the environment have seen the emergence of new interdisciplinary fields; yet the feasibility of the paradigm in the wake of managed care is questionable.

Summary

The behavioral medicine paradigm is based on the premise that physical problems are related to lifestyle and an individual's interaction with the environment (Raines & Erickson, 1997). The paradigm depends upon careful analysis of all factors in relation to the etiology and maintenance of health (Pinkerton et al., 1982). The most important factor in developing a behavioral modification strategy is individualized assessment of the behavior that is to be changed (Wodarski et al., 1991).

Health Belief Model

The Health Belief Model was first developed in the 1950s by social psychologists at the United States Public Health Service (Hochbaum, 1958; Rosenstock & Kirscht, 1974). The model was developed in an effort to explain the reasons for the widespread failure of people to participate in prevention programs. This model was later extended to apply to an individual's response to health related symptoms as well as responses to diagnosed illness and compliance with medical regimens (Rosenstock, 1990). The Health Belief Model has become one of the most influential and widely used approaches to explaining health related behavior (Rosenstock, 1990). The model focuses on cognitive influences of behavior (Kaplan et al., 1993).

Assumptions

1   Efficacy exceptions (Rosenstock, 1990). It is believed that individuals will take action to ward off, to screen for or control ill health conditions if they believe themselves to be susceptible to the illness (Rosenstock, 1990). The individual will also take action if he/she believes the illness to have serious consequences, if the course of action available would reduce his/her susceptibility to the illness or if the benefits are seen to outweigh the costs. The perceived benefits and perceived barriers are considered together in a cost–benefit analysis (Kaplan et al., 1993). There are many different variables that contribute to the Health Belief Model such as perceptions of susceptibility, severity, benefits, barriers, and demographic variable.

2   Self-efficacy plays a large role in the Health Belief Model by giving it an increased explanatory power. According to Rosenstock (1990) outcome expectation is similar to the Health Belief Model's concept of perceived benefits. Self-efficacy is the "conviction that one can successfully execute the behavior required to produce the outcomes" (Bandura, 1977, p. 79). Perceived benefits determine the actions an individual will take depending on the feasibility and the efficaciousness of the recommended health action. Reviews of the Health Belief Model have provided substantial empirical support for the model (Rosenstock, 1990). In 1984, Janz and Becker reviewed twenty-nine studies of the Health Belief Model as well as tabulating the findings of seventeen studies conducted prior to 1974. The researchers also provided summaries of all forty-six Health Belief Model studies. Eighteen of the studies were prospective and twenty-eight were retrospective. The findings indicated that the findings from the prospective studies were at least as favorable as the retrospective (Rosenstock, 1990).

Critiques

The Health Belief Model is not without its critiques. One criticism holds that the belief-behavior relationship has never been established. Behavior cannot always be accounted for by beliefs (Rosenstock, 1990), yet beliefs often account for the variance in behavior. People do not live in a vacuum. There are often many psychological factors that play a role in the formation of behaviors (Rosenstock, 1990). Researchers need to take this fact into account and not dismiss the model entirely.

A second criticism is that oftentimes direct attempts to modify are unsuccessful and alternative approaches are necessary (Rosenstock, 1990). This criticism is perplexing in that the model is not intended to be utilized as a strategy for change. In addition, environmental and structural changes may have an effect on health belief (Rosenstock & Kirscht, 1974).

Those who defend the Health Belief Model state that it is usually possible to assign blame without the help of a model (Rosenstock, 1990). In the case of the Health Belief Model, victim blaming is not the issue in as much as the client is taking responsibility for solving the problem, the crux of behavioral medicine (Rosenstock, 1990).

Summary

The Health Belief Model was developed to explain the failure of individuals to participate in preventive medicine. The model is one of the most influential approaches to explaining health-related behaviors. The main assumptions of the model are that the three main components are threat, expectations and efficacy, and expectations with self-efficacy. Criticisms include the failure of the model to establish belief–behavior relationship, the need for alternative approaches to modify behavior, lack of quantification, and blaming the victim.

Theory of Reasoned Action

The Theory of Reasoned Action (Fishbein, 1967) describes the interplay between belief, attitudes, intentions, and behavior. The theory attempts to predict a person's intention to perform a behavior in a particular setting. The theory assumes that intention is the immediate determinant of behavior.

Assumptions

1 People are generally rational and make predictable use of the information available to them (Kaplan et al., 1993).
2 All factors that influence behavior are mediated through intention (Carter, 1990).
3 The strengths of an individual's intention to perform a behavior are the function of two factors: attitude toward the behavior and the influence of the environment.

4   Attitude toward behavior is determined by an individual's belief that a given outcome will occur if he or she performs the behavior and by an evaluation of the outcome (Carter, 1990).

5   Subjective norms, sometimes called social norms, are the individual's perceptions of social influences about performing the behavior (Kaplan et al., 1993).

6   Attitudes and subjective norms determine intentions regarding a behavior. Subjective norms are those that are most likely to be affected by pressure from significant others.

Critique

Although the Theory of Reasoned Action does provide a framework providing insight into underlying reasons for action or non-action in terms of health, it does not take into account diversity of population (Montano et al., 1997), such as race or socioeconomic status. Race and socioeconomic status play a role in explaining people's behaviors, especially in terms of health care. These factors need to be taken into account to have a more accurate explanation of an individual's behavior. The Theory of Reasoned Action does not specify the particular beliefs about behavioral outcomes that should be measures. These beliefs may be difficult for the same behavior among different populations (Montano et al., 1997).

Summary

The Theory of Reasoned Action is based on the premise that there is interplay between attitude, intention, and behavior. The major assumption of the theory is that all factors that influence behavior are mediated through intentions. There are underlying reasons determining an individual's motivation to perform a behavior. The theory does not, however, take into account diversity of individuals in terms of race or socioeconomic status.

Multi-attribute Utility Theory

The Multi-attribute Utility Theory predicts behavior from an individual's evaluation of the outcomes or consequences associated with performing and not performing a specific behavior (Carter, 1990). This theory provides a methodology for breaking down complex decisions into individual attributes that may influence a decision. The theory also provides a methodology for having the individual make a decision by evaluating each attribute, as well as the methodology for combining the evaluations into an overall score in order to predict the course of action the individual is likely to take (Carter, 1990).

Application

The Multi-attribute Utility Theory has been applied to important related decisions (Beach et al., 1976). This application is utilized to achieve one or both of two goals:

1 To spur the development of interventions designed to influence decision.
2 Provide a vehicle to aid in decision making.

The information for the Multi-attribute Utility Theory model surrounding consequences or outcomes has been obtained empirically from explanatory interviews with a representative sample (Carter, 1990). The content of this theory is dependent on the information elicited from these interviews.

Critique

Both the Theory of Reasoned Action and the Multi-attribute Utility Theory are diagnostic in that they describe the issues and concerns of differentiate individuals who have accomplished behavior change and those who have not (Carter, 1990). Prochaska and DeClemente (1983) suggest that it is useful to use the process mentioned above while broadening the perspective of individual decision making.

Summary

The two primary applications are to spur development of decisions to influence decisions and to provide a vehicle to aid in decision making. This theory only offers a snapshot of how personal decisions are made. A combination of the Multi-attribute Utility Theory and a broad perspective on decision making is needed to understand personal decision making.

Social Cognitive Theory

Social Cognitive Theory is a theory that addresses the psychosocial issues underlying health behaviors as well as promoting behavior change.

Assumptions

The Social Cognitive Theory is based on the following assumptions:

1 Behavior, personal factors and environmental influences all interact.
2 Environmental factors play an important role in today's illness.

3   The basic social cognitive techniques of respondent and operant conditioning, which operate on environmental influences, are choice treatments in behavioral medicine (Pinkerton et al., 1982).
4   The base of Social Cognitive Theory is grounded in the conditioning theories, which state that learning occurs through prior experiences. The behavior is usually influenced by its consequences (Bandura, 1977).

Albert Bandura is the leading figure in the understanding of the relationship of cognitive constructs in Social Cognitive Theory. In 1969, Bandura provided a framework for behavioral modification that emphasized the traditional learning theory. Social Cognitive Theory employs many constructs that are important in the understanding of human behavior. The constructs of Social Cognitive Theory include the environment, expectations, situations, behavioral capabilities, self-control, observational learning, reinforcements, self-efficacy, coping responses, and reciprocal determinism. All of these constructs allow for the understanding of human behavior and the implications for behavioral change. Social Cognitive Theory highlights the dynamics of an individual's behavior and gives direction as to the intervention strategies to facilitate behavioral change.

Summary

The Social Cognitive Theory is based on the premise that behavior, personal factors and environment all interact, with the environment playing a role in illness. The theory is based on many constructs, all of which allow for the understanding of human behavior and the implications for behavioral change. Critics of the theory feel that it may be too comprehensive and have too many constructs. It is important for supporters of the theory to be very specific in identifying the phenomenon and only report empirical evidence.

Trans-theoretical Model

The Trans-theoretical Model was developed by Prochaska, Norcross, and DeClemente (1994). Their observations led to the notion that people appear to go through similar stages of change no matter the therapy. The model suggests that different intervention approaches are needed for people at different stages of change but also which processes are most important at each stage.

Prochaska (1996) suggests that the stage paradigm involves change as a six-stage process:

1   Pre-contemplation: People are not intending to take action within the near future. Individuals in this stage are typically defensive and resistant. Some are demoralized by past failures.

2   Contemplation: People are intending to take action in the near future. Individuals are aware of the benefits of change, as well as the costs of change.
3   Preparation: People are ready to participate in action oriented interventions. Motivation is key.
4   Action: Involves overt behavioral modification. Hard work usually lasts for six months.
5   Maintenance: Continue to apply process of change, yet do not have to work as hard. Common time for relapse. Some will remain in this stage for the rest of their lives.
6   Termination: Period of no longer having to apply processes of change. Some never reach this stage.

The Trans-theoretical Model follows the following set of assumptions (Prochaska et al., 1997):

1   No single theory can account for the complexities of behavioral change.
2   Behavioral change is a process that unfolds over time through stages.
3   Stages are stable and open to change.
4   Without planned interventions populations will remain stuck in the early stages.
5   The majority of at risk populations are not prepared for action.
6   Specific processes and principles of change need to be applied at certain stages to initiate change.
7   Chronic behavioral patterns are a combination of biology, social influences, and self-control.

Critique

The Trans-theoretical Model is based on the premise that individuals are in one of six stages of change, based on their readiness to change. Different interventions are needed at each stage of change. The main assumptions of the Trans-theoretical Model are based on the idea that no single theory can explain behavioral change and that all individuals go through stages when trying to engage in behavioral change and these stages are stable yet open to change. Without planned interventions at each stage, individuals will become stuck in one stage and will not be able to obtain the desired behavioral change.

Summary

Theory helps in the selection of appropriate interventions by delineating the what, how, when and why of behavior (Glanz et al., 1990). There is no single theory that explains human behavior in terms of prevention of disease. The behavioral medicine paradigm depends on an individual's lifestyle, and the interactions with their social environment (Pinkerton et al., 1982). This paradigm replaces the single cause of disease model of causation of disease (McClelland, 1989). Consequently, new fields have emerged such as psychobiology, sociobiology and behavioral medicine, breaking the traditional boundaries between fields (Wodarski et al., 1991).

Many models and theories have been applied to help explain the field of behavioral medicine. These models include the Health Belief Model, Theory of Reasoned Action, Multi-attribute Utility Theory, Social Cognitive Theory, and Trans-theoretical Model.

Adult Interventions

A variety of interventions have been utilized to treat chronic diseases. This section outlines behavioral techniques used to treat chronic diseases. The section also delineates the various behavioral interventions used to treat some of the more common chronic diseases and issues among women. These interventions include respondent and operant techniques, cognitive procedures, integrated interventions, and interventions for specific risk factors such as hypertension, inactivity, and smoking. Operant techniques and cognitive procedures have been described in detail in Chapter 1. This section provides examples of behavioral techniques specific to adult diseases.

Respondent Techniques

Respondent behaviors—also known as Pavlonian Behaviors—are those elicited by preceding stimuli and involve an involuntary response or reflex (Baldwin & Baldwin, 1986). These involuntary responses may include salivation response to food, or an increased heart rate in response to stress. Most unconditioned reflexes have a positive or negative emotional component. Respondent conditioning occurs when after repeated pairings, a neutral stimulus acquires the eliciting properties of the original stimulus (Wodarski et al., 1991). In terms of behavioral medicine, stress is a significant factor. For example, if work produces many stressful events, eventually simply going to work will become stressful.

Relaxation

Relaxation is typically defined in one of two ways. Davidson and Schwartz (1976a) define a relaxation response as being low physiological arousal. The "specificity model," defined by Davidson and Schwartz (1976a; 1976b; 1976c), differentiates between cognitive, somatic, and behavioral relaxation. In this case, cognitive relaxation (meditation) is used for cognitive symptoms such as worry, while somatic treatments such as progressive relaxation are utilized for somatic symptoms (Smith et al., 1996). Relaxation should be considered a general coping skill. It can be used as a counter to specific stressors or as a general strategy to prevent negative reactions to stress (Watson & Tharp, 1993).

Application

Relaxation is commonly used in pairing with physiological hyper-arousal symptoms (Blanchard et al., 1989). Relaxation can be used to reduce anxiety experienced in a particular situation, prior to re-experiencing the situation. The most frequent problem in developing a relaxation program is simply not doing it, particularly in the early stages (Watson & Tharp, 1993). Some common excuses for non-compliance with a relaxation program are having no place to relax, the program seems boring, and not having enough time.

Systematic Desensitization

Systematic desensitization is a procedure in which the individual imagines the anxiety-producing situation. The individual then breaks the situation down into a series of steps, progressing from the lowest to highest anxiety-producing (Wodarski & Bagarozzi, 1979).

Counter-Conditioning

Counter-conditioning is a technique in which the stimulus that produces a maladaptive response is paired with a response that is incompatible with the maladaptive response. For example, cancer patients who are undergoing chemotherapy often experience nausea and vomiting. Over time, the patients may develop a conditioned response to which simply entering the treatment office results in the individual becoming nauseous (Wodarski et al., 1991).

Aversive Counter-Conditioning

Aversive counter-conditioning is the pairing of a maladaptive positive response with aversive stimuli. Gradually, the maladaptive response loses its attractiveness and becomes either neutral or aversive (Baldwin & Baldwin, 1986). In other words, when the problem and the emotion are paired with aversive stimuli, the problem is no longer attractive.

Integrated Intervention

Clinical interventions typically have the highest efficacy rate in terms of behavioral change, but do not reach many individuals (Prochaska, 1996). Conversely, public health interventions have the highest reach, but the lowest efficacy. It would then seem logical to attempt to combine the two approaches to offer the best possible interventions while reaching as many individuals as possible (Prochaska, 1996).

Prochaska (1996) suggests applying this stage paradigm to the most important phases of planned intervention: Recruitment, Retention, Progress, Process, and Outcomes. Prochaska (1996) suggests proactive rather than reactive recruitment techniques. Retention, progress, and process are all assessed based on the stage of change the individual is demonstrating. The matching of interventions are based on a participant's needs rather than on the needs of the program (Prochaska, 1996).

Cardiovascular Disease

Cardiovascular Disorders

Cardiovascular and renal diseases account for a large proportion of adult deaths in the United States (Shapiro & Goldstein, 1982). Hypertension is a major risk factor for the development of these diseases. The maintenance of high blood pressure over long periods of time increases the likelihood of damaging the heart, blood vessels, and kidneys.

Essentially, hypertension is of greater interest to those in behavioral medicine because it is often not associated with a specific physical cause. While there is a genetic predisposition for the development of hypertension, approximately 70 percent of its etiology may be due to environmental factors (Weiner, 1979). Drug therapy is commonly used in the treatment of hypertension. As Shapiro and Goldstein (1982) point out, however, drug therapy does not treat the underlying causes. The physical risk factors which are most often the target of behavioral treatment efforts are dietary restrictions, such as the reduction of sodium intake (Pickering, 1982), weight loss (Eliahou et al., 1981), and regular exercise (Horton, 1981). Others have examined these risk factors in combination. Stamler et al. (1980), for example, reported data that suggests that a nutritional information program combined with exercise can benefit both those who already have essential hypertension and those who are at high risk for its development.

Hypertension

Hypertension affects over 60 million individuals in the United States (Eisenberg et al., 1993, Weaver & McGrady, 1995). If uncontrolled, hypertension can lead to renal disease, stroke, myocardio infarction, congestive heart failure, and coronary artery disease. Hypertension has been the most frequently reported morbidity related diagnosis in National Surveys since 1973 (Eisenberg et al., 1993). Hypertension is primarily treated with the use of anti-hypertensive medications. Medications do indeed lower the blood pressure of the individual, yet do nothing to address the underlying causes of what has lead to the elevation in blood pressure (Wodarski et al., 1991). Though genetics, race, and gender play a strong role in the development on hypertension (McGrady & Roberts, 1992; Roberts & McGrady, 1996), there is strong evidence to suggest that most often, hypertension is caused by environmental or behavioral factors. These behavioral factors include dietary fat intake, sodium intake, exercise, and stress.

There is rising evidence on the association between job stress and physical health of workers (Bosma et al., 1998). Persons in high strain jobs are at a higher risk of coronary heart disease. High job strain results when the demands of the job are high and a worker's sense of control over the work is low (Sorensen et al., 1996). Low job control has been found to increase the risk of coronary heart disease. Similarly, a high effort–reward imbalance has also been shown to be related to coronary heart disease (Bosma et al. 1998). Sorensen et al. (1996) found that blood pressure is higher among men than among women and increases with education.

In a sex specific study, "unemployment, worry about losing one's job, and feeling less than very good at doing one's job" were predictors of hypertension among the male population. Among the female population, "anomy and depressive symptoms" were predictors for the disease. In both male and female sexes, "low education, African American race, and low occupational status" were predictors of hypertension (Levenstein et al., 2001).

As mentioned above, cardiovascular disease is the leading cause of death among adults. This section outlines the various behavioral techniques utilized to treat one type of cardiovascular disease: hypertension.

Biofeedback

Biofeedback is the feeding back of physiological activity. This feeding back is done with audio or visual devices that allow the patient to gain an awareness of what is happening inside his or her body (Eisenberg et al., 1993). A person can be trained to control blood pressure, blood flow, heart rate, and skin temperature. Patients are trained to decrease forehead muscle tension and increase finger temperature. This method has also been used as a method to lower stress levels, consequently lowering blood pressure (McGrady & Roberts, 1992).

Studies have shown that 50–80 percent of individuals with hypertension, treated with biofeedback, lowered their blood pressure by a significant amount, while 20–30 percent showed no improvement (Blanchard et al., 1991; Fahrion et al., 1986; Glasgow et al., 1982; Patel & North, 1975). When used alone, biofeedback did little to add to the practice of relaxation. Biofeedback has the greatest success when combined with other forms of relaxation, exercise, and a healthy diet (Lehrer et al., 1994).

Relaxation Training

Transcendental meditation has reduced several risk factors of cardiovascular disease, including hypertension, in clinical studies (Zamarra et al., 1996). Studies have suggested that a lower rate of cardiovascular morbidity and mortality have been associated with long term practice of transcendental meditation (Orme-Johnson, 1987). Though drug therapies tend to be most effective in lowering blood pressure, several studies have revealed that stress management techniques are effective for people with mild hypertension. This allows for a lesser dosage of medication (Lehrer et al., 1994).

The word "stress" is derived from the Latin meaning "to draw together tightly." When the individual is experiencing stress, the mind tightens, narrowing perceptions and decreasing options for maintaining homeostasis (Arnold, 1997).

The influence of stress on various diseases, particularly hypertension, has become increasingly prominent in recent years (Lehrer et al., 1994). Consequently, stress management techniques are becoming more accepted practices among health care workers. The enormous cost associated with the treatment of hypertension coupled with the increasing attention given to quality of life and adherence issues has spurred the exploration of behavioral techniques in treatment (Weaver & McGrady, 1995). Linden and Chambers (1994) have suggested that non-drug therapies may be more effective than previously believed. These stress management techniques include biofeedback, relaxation training, and meditation.

Stress Management

An awareness of the differential impact of various emotional states on cardiovascular functioning has implications as an adjunct to stress management training. Stress management is a strategy that attempts to minimize the effect a person's daily stresses have on their blood pressure. Stress management training can be conducted either in groups or individually (Roskies, 1987). The aim is to remove, reduce, and/or neutralize the stresses within the individual's environment (Wodarski & Wodarski, 1993).

For many years, autonomic emotional responses have been thought to function as links between psychological functioning and proneness to physical diseases (Schwartz et al., 1981). Schwartz et al. examined the effect that various emotions (happiness, sadness, anger, and fear) have on the cardio-vascular system. Data produced evidence of specific patterns of cardiovascular adjustments that are evoked by each of these emotions. Anger was found to have a much greater effect on the cardiovascular system than any of the other emotions. This effect was opposite to that of relaxation. These authors comment that this is consistent with "evidence of the special role of hostility in hypertension and cardiovascular disease" (p. 358).

As Schwartz et al. (1981) point out, the emotional responses meditate differentially between environmental stress and cardiovascular responses. The impact which sadness was found to have is especially interesting because it interfered with the cardiovascular adjustments which are normally produced by exercise. This illustrates the power of the link between the emotions and cardiovascular functioning. This linkage and the differential meditation process is important for the helping professional to understand so that this knowledge can be incorporated into the prevention and treatment of cardiovascular disorders. Future conceptualizations will emphasize a multi-component model (Byrne, 1989a, 1989b; Contrada, 1989).

Exercise

Regular exercise can reduce the impact of stressful life events in terms of the prevalence of an illness (Packard, 2005; Shepard, 1997; Winerman, 2005). Roth and Holmes (1987) found that students who had a low level of physical activity became ill more often upon the introduction of stressful events. Individuals with a moderate or high level of fitness were more protected against illnesses. In a similar study, Folkins and Sime (1981) found that in patients who are depressed, physical exercise such as running proved to be just as effective in relieving the depression as psychotherapy.

Inactivity

The American Heart Association has added inactivity to its list of modifiable risk factors (Anderson et al., 1998). Yet only 22 percent of the American adult populations is active enough to derive health benefits. One of the results of inactivity, obesity, can lead to many potentially serious conditions.

Obesity

Obesity is a life threatening disorder associated with many co-morbid conditions and leads to an impaired quality of life (Pekkarinen & Mustajoki,

1997). Excess body weight is associated with hypertension, diabetes, and hyper-cholesterolemia. It is also a risk factor of coronary heart disease and some cancers (Lewis et al., 1997).

Obesity develops from an imbalance between the amount of energy intake and the amount of energy expended (Lewis et al., 1997). Obesity is a multi-determined condition that depends on both genetics and behavior to develop. Though genetics play a role in obesity, it is little disputed that the development of obesity is largely dependent upon individual behaviors (Lewis et al., 1997). People who are obese eat more than those who are not obese (Drougas et al., 1992; Heitmann, 1993; Lichtman et al., 1992; Livingstone et al., 1990; Maffeis et al., 1994; Schoeller, 1990).

Obesity Consequence

While there is widespread agreement that gross obesity directly endangers one's health, the danger is less clear for persons who are less than 30 percent overweight (Brownell, 1982a). However, obesity does endanger one's health indirectly by increasing the likelihood of developing hypertension, hyper-lipemia, and diabetes (Andres, 1980; Keys, 1980).

Brownell and Wadden (1986) report that more than one hundred controlled studies have been conducted on the social learning treatment of obesity. Social learning weight loss programs have repeatedly produced positive results (Stalonas et al., 1984) and have demonstrated short-term maintenance of these results (Jeffery et al., 1978; Mahoney, 1974a, 1974b, 1974c, 1974d; Stalonas et al., 1978). Aversive therapy and covert sensitization were sometimes used in the past, but their largely negative results have discouraged their usage (Abramson, 1977).

In his review of social learning approaches to the treatment of obesity, Abramson (1973) concluded that self-control procedures are the most promising. These procedures are of two types: complex and simple self-control. Complex self-control "involves self monitoring, cognitive imagery of expectations and body image, self-reinforcement, and stimulus control techniques intended to reduce the number of environmental stimuli that trigger eating" (Abramson, 1977, p. 357). These treatments have produced largely positive results.

Exercise plays an important role in both the prevention and treatment of obesity. Exercise is advocated for health improvement because it burns calories, yet the long-term cumulative effects are more important for health improvement than are the short term caloric expenditures (Brownell, 1982a, 1982b, 1982c; Craighead & Blum, 1989). Exercise is able to counteract obesity's negative effects by its positive influence on plasma insulin levels, blood pressure, and coronary efficiency, even in the absence of weight loss

(Bjorntorp, 1978; Bray, 1976; Brownell et al., 1980; Scheurer & Tipton, 1977). Exercise also aids in weight loss by suppressing the appetite and by offsetting the decline in basal metabolic rate which is created by dieting (Brownell, 1982a).

Regular exercise is important for other aspects of health as well. Aerobic exercise aids in the prevention and/or treatment of a variety of disorders (Martin & Dubbert, 1982). Exercise programs have been used extensively in both the prevention and treatment of heart disease. Systematic aerobic exercise has been shown to improve cardiovascular efficiency (Scheurer & Tipton, 1977) and to modify cardiovascular risk profiles in healthy individuals, those at risk for coronary disease, and coronary patients (Clausen, 1976; Kannel & Sorlie, 1979; Leon & Blackburn, 1977; Mann et al., 1969; Wilhelmsen et al., 1975).

Exercise is also helpful in the behavioral management of diabetes (Martin & Dubbert, 1982). Regular exercise is recommended for diabetics as a part of their treatment, due to its potential to improve metabolic control, to reduce plasma insulin, to improve insulin sensitivity, and to improve glucose tolerance (Soman et al., 1979).

Attrition is a tremendous problem with exercise programs. Studies show that half or less of the individuals who begin an exercise program will be in that program for three to six months (Durbeck et al., 1972; Taylor et al., 1973). This is true for both self-initiated programs and structured programs. Staying in an exercise program may be even more difficult for smokers (Clark et al., 1996).

Exercise programs should be designed with attention given to the fact that most attrition occurs in the early stages of participation. Adaptations may be necessary for individuals who are at high risk for dropping out. Martin and Dubbert (1982) suggest that it may be necessary to begin with a single exercise, establish it in a single environment, and then extend it to other environments (stimulus generalization). They state that other exercise behaviors can then be established in the same way (in a single environment first).

It is important to address expectations as well. Exercise programs should be tailored to the individual in such a way that the goals established are small and realistic. Danielson and Wanzel (1977) found that those who did not achieve their own goals dropped out at twice the rate of those who were successful with small and realistic goals. This suggests that the sense of achievement created by the attainment of small goals will do much to encourage the exerciser to continue in his or her efforts.

Comprehensive programs are necessary that focus on multiple variables which affect weight loss, such as genetic factors, nutrition, exercise, social support, metabolic rate, and socioeconomic status (Van Itallie, 1986).

Exercise

The relationship between activity level and obesity is well researched (Clark et al., 1996). People who are obese exercise less than individuals who are lean. Exercise plays a crucial role in both the prevention and treatment of obesity. Exercise lowers blood pressure, reduces risk of coronary artery disease and hypertension, lowers depression and anxiety levels, and augments weight loss (Fletcher et al., 1995).

The Center for Disease Control and the American College of Sports Medicine suggest that all Americans should exercise at least thirty minutes every day (Andersen et al., 1998). Reports suggest that only 22 percent of the United States adult population are active enough for any health benefits. In addition, it is estimated that one of every four Americans is completely sedentary (U.S. Public Health Service, 1996).

Worksite Interventions

Worksites offer opportunities to encourage adults and their families to increase activity levels (Dishman et al., 1998). Europe pioneered the worksite intervention movement (Sallis et al., 1998). The worksite intervention studies eliminated traditional barriers to exercise (Storer et al., 1997). Results of worksite interventions have not been statistically significant. No more than 30 percent of employees participated and only 50 percent of those maintained the exercise. The percentages are even lower for blue collar employees (Storer et al., 1997).

There are two possible explanations for the limited impact of the worksite interventions (Storer et al., 1997). First, is that education restructuring and behavioral modification efforts were not successful. A second explanation is that the factors identified in the health behavioral model are necessary conditions for changing health behaviors. The components of the Health Belief Model are perception of susceptibility, severity, benefits, and barriers. The model implies the weighting of these perceptions as the motivation for health behavior change (Storer et al., 1997). There have been few worksite intervention studies that have utilized valid research designs and measures (Dishman et al., 1998).

Community Interventions

In the early 1980s Brownell and colleagues (1980) studied the effects of placing signs encouraging stair use at the base of an escalator that was adjacent to stairs. The sign resulted in statistically significant increases in stair use. Blamey et al. (1995) conducted a study in an attempt to increase stair use in a subway station. The intervention consisted of posting a sign for three weeks that said: "Stay healthy, save time, use the stairs." Stair use increased from 5 percent to 12 percent for women and from 12 percent to 21 percent for men.

Andersen et al. (1998) investigated the stair and elevator use trends among shoppers of different ages, ethnicity, sex, and body types in a shopping mall. The researchers observed the effects of adding signs at the base of the escalator promoting stair use. Two signs were used at different times. One sign featured a picture of a heart and read "Your heart needs exercise, use the stairs" (Andersen et al., 1998, p. 364). The second signal had a picture of a woman with a small waistline wearing pants that were too big. The sign read "Improve your waistline, use the stairs" (Andersen et al., 1998, p. 364). The researchers found that visual cues emphasizing weight control were as effective if not more so than signs highlighting health benefits. Older people increased stair use regardless of the sign used.

These studies indicate that cost-effective interventions significantly increase physical activity. Andersen et al. (1998) estimated the cost of placing one sign in each shopping mall in the United States to be $110,000 at a rate of $60 per sign. For a sign to be placed in each shopping mall in the United States, this would result in more than 1.6 million Americans using the stairs instead of an escalator. The caloric cost of walking up and down two flights of stairs every day would amount to an average weight loss of 2.7kg for the average man (Brownell et al., 1980).

Behavioral Interventions

The behavioral changes necessary to achieve weight loss and maintain the loss are very difficult for most people who are obese (Jeffery & French, 1997). People who are obese tend to restrict their dietary intake during the day and then overeat in the evening hours succumbing to their hunger (Clark et al., 1996). It is important that questions about the number of meals consumed in a day and the types of snacks eaten in a day be asked by the researcher when conducting a weight loss intervention (Clark et al., 1996), so as to develop an appropriate strategy for each individual.

In order to effectively help an individual treat his or her obesity, it is important to assess the degree of desire for change. As mentioned above, individuals move through stages of change. The preparation stage is where intervention is crucial. These individuals are ready to begin the process of change (Prochaska et al., 1994). The action stage is the time of dieting and exercise intervention. The individual is committed to change.

Many obese patients seen in the primary change setting are in the pre-contemplation and contemplation stages (Clark et al., 1996). In a 1992 survey, only 53 percent of obese adults were willing to attempt to lose weight. Almost 50 percent were not taking action (Kuczmarski & Flegal, 1994). Though this percentage is discouraging, all hope is not lost. Primary physicians have more influence on their patient's weight management than they realize. In a survey conducted by Levy and Williamson (1988), 81 percent of those who were currently trying to lose weight, or already had lost weight, had been informed by a physician that they were overweight. Brief intervention by physicians may have significant effects on a patient's motivation to lose weight.

Smoking

The use of tobacco has significantly declined over the past couple of decades, yet smoking still remains the leading cause of premature death in the United States (U.S. Department of Health, 1994). Tobacco use is the single most preventable cause of death, yet is responsible for 30 percent of all cancer deaths, and 87 percent of all lung cancer deaths (U.S. Department of Health, 1991). Cigarette smoking has been proven to be a major risk factor in heart disease, cancers, and stroke. Even with this being the case, approximately 29 percent of the United States population smoke tobacco (Elixhauser, 1990).

Most smokers have reported that they have seriously considered quitting, yet in actuality, almost 40 percent of people who are currently smoking are not considering quitting (Curry et al., 1997).

The key factor in smoking cessation is motivation (Curry et al., 1997). In the case of cigarette smoking, motivation refers to both the level of the individual's desire to quit as well as the type of motivation (Curry et al., 1997). Assessing and enhancing motivation is a challenge for those in the behavioral health field, as well as for those in the medical field (Curry et al., 1997). This challenge is magnified by the reluctance of primary physicians, chemical dependency clinicians, and psychiatrists to address issues of smoking cessation (Hughes, 1996). One possible reason for the reluctance may be the intrinsic belief that smokers choose to quit on their own, with success. The fact that smoking involves a nicotine dependence is often ignored (Hughes, 1996).

The majority of smoking cessation literature has a strong behavioral focus (Wodarski et al., 1991). There is, however, evidence that there is a group of regular smokers who are highly addicted (Curry et al., 1997), and in items of cessation, this group is having very little success (Hughes, 1996).

The number of women smoking increased dramatically during and after World War II, with women reporting a greater tendency to cut back rather than quit (Whitlock et al., 1997).

Smoking Consequences

The U.S. Surgeon General (U.S. DHEW, 1979) reports the three leading causes of death in the U.S. are heart disease, malignant neoplasms, and stroke. Cigarette smoking is a proven major risk factor in all three of these causes of death (Lichtenstein, 1982). Smoking has received a tremendous amount of attention in recent years. The smoking cessation literature is extensive with most of its focus on behavioral work, the majority of which has been directed at control, rather than prevention.

Smoking is one strategy for coping with stress. The smoking ritual may become a coping response through response generalization (Pomerleau, 1981). Several studies, such as the one by McRae and Choi-Lao (1978), have linked anxiety to smoking behavior. Williams et al. (1982) administered the MMPI's Manifest Anxiety Scale to fifty smokers and fifty nonsmokers. The mean scores of the smokers were significantly higher than those of the non-smokers, and significantly more smokers had physical symptoms related to anxiety than did the non-smokers.

Although various methods report short-term success at bringing about smoking cessation, long-term abstinence rates are generally poor. An exception is Lando and McGovern (1982), who followed subjects from a study by Lando (1981). At 12, 18, 24, and 36 months, subjects who had received a two-stage (aversion and maintenance) intensive contact treatment exhibited a consistent abstinence of 40 percent.

Most of the behavioral treatments for smoking cessation are multi-component. Almost always included are self-control procedures, stimulus control, and the development of substitute behaviors for smoking (Lichtenstein & Mermelstein, 1986). They elaborate that other behaviors, such as relaxation training, stress management, or contingency contracting, may be included as well.

More research is needed on the differences between smokers who are able to quit and smokers who are not. The major difference may be the cognitive expectations of individuals who believe that they can stop (Yates & Thain, 1985). For those who have great difficulty in quitting, controlled smoking may be the best alternative. In controlled smoking, smokers are trained to reduce their CO levels by such instructions as "take shorter puffs" or "take six puffs less on each cigarette" (Frederiksen & Simon, 1978a, 1978b). Stitzer and Bigelow (1985) also did a study which reviews examined CO levels. They demonstrated that contingent reinforcement, based on CO levels in expiration, can exercise target-specific control over smoking behavior.

Smoking behavior should be examined in the context of an individual's total health behavior. Kristiansen (1985) surveyed 113 persons and found that the smoking item was correlated with the total preventative health behavior scores. Other studies, such as Eiser and Sutton (1979), have reported that smokers exhibit more health protective behaviors than non-smokers.

A logical and convenient location for smoking cessation services is as the worksite. Businesses are becoming increasingly concerned about the health of their employees, and thus are giving more attention to the promotion of wellness behaviors, such as smoking cessation.

Smoking Cessation

As in the case with obesity, a review of the literature indicates that there are positive results when primary care physicians intercede with their parents who smoke. The use of primary care physician as educator, facilitator, and counselor has great potential to have a drastic impact on smoking cessation (Ockene & Zapka, 1997). Studies have demonstrated that the stronger the physician intervention, the greater effect smoking cessation was found in the condition where the physician spent most of the time with the patient. In addition to the amount of time spent with a patient, randomized trials have found that multiple intervention components have a greater success rate that single interventions (Ockene & Zapka, 1997). Five trials have been funded by the National Cancer Institute, all using some form of physician intervention. The three successful trials, however, demonstrated that a second intervention was utilized. This intervention was in the form of a reminder system, and in one trial phone counseling (Ockene & Zapka, 1997).

Despite the positive results of these interventions, many primary physicians do not address smoking cessation and possible interventions (Richmond et al., 1998). This failure to address smoking is often due to the fact that primary physicians have little training in treating individuals who smoke and they see smoking as being a complex subject to counsel patients about (Hughes, 1996). Physicians are more likely to provide cessation interventions if they have training on the subject (Richmond et al., 1998). Education of health care providers that builds knowledge, confidence and skills must occur in the context of multi-model interventions in the physician office (Ockene & Zapka, 1997). The utilization of smoking cessation interventions by family physicians was assessed by Richmond et al. (1998). Ninety-three percent of the physicians reported that a workshop gave them sufficient training and only 14 percent reported a lack of confidence in administering the program. Eighty-eight percent of the physicians reported the program at a six-month follow up. The effect of reinforcement health care settings has the potential to provide opportunities to reach tobacco users with personalized cessation interventions (Lichtenstein et al., 1996). Health care settings provide the opportunity to reach populations of smokers by combining public health and clinical approaches to smoking cessation. Five key issues must be addressed when implementing cessation in health care facilities (Lichtenstein et al., 1996):

1 Investigators must decide on whether to focus on physicians or to adopt an approach utilizing other personnel.
2 Choices made with respect to length and intensity of counseling.
3 The extent of tailoring to the patient's readiness to quit as well as attention to the psychosocial factors.
4 Emphasis on behavioral vs. pharmacological approaches.
5 Efficacy trial vs. effectiveness trial.

Following a low intensity intervention at large Health Management Organizations (HMO) that utilized messages, videos, carbon monoxide tests and feedback to the patient, the quit rate was modest, yet doubled that of the advice only condition (Hollis et al., 1993).

Hospital-based Interventions

Hospitalization may provide an opportune time to change smoking behavior simply because it requires smokers to abstain (Rigotti et al., 1997). During hospitalization, many patients will temporarily lose interest in smoking due to the illness (Lichtenstein et al., 1996).

Past research suggests that a hospital stay can trigger cessation. In one study, 16 percent of patients who smoked at the time of admission were no longer smoking one year later. The annual smoking cessation rate is approximately 7 percent. A higher cessation rate has been reported by smokers with smoking related diseases (Rigotti et al., 1997). Stevens et al. (1993) found that after an intervention consisting of bedside counseling and telephone follow up after discharge, 13.5 percent of the patients had quit smoking as opposed to 9.2 percent in the usual care group. This research suggests that hospitalization provides yet another "teachable moment" (Lichtenstein et al., 1996, p. 715) of a captive audience.

Mass Media Interventions

Mass media has the potential to be a powerful intervention that can be applied in a positive manner. Mass media interventions typically used for smoking cessation include posters, billboards, videos, television, and radio. The most effective interventions are placed where people are more likely to be reached (Ruiter et al., 2006).

Mass media may be an effective way to decrease cigarette smoking (Goldman & Glantz, 1998). The effectiveness of mass media in decreasing cigarette smoking in adults and children was assessed and it was found that aggressiveness and a focus on second-hand smoke to be the most effective approaches. A second finding was that teens often initiated smoking as a means of showing autonomy. Due to this quest for autonomy, mass media directed at teens is most effective when demonstrating how tobacco companies use advertising to coerce adolescents to smoke. The teens that are trying to rebel begin to see that they are actually doing what the tobacco companies want them to do (Goldman & Glantz, 1998).

Mass media interventions can help enhance the effectiveness of school smoking prevention programs (Worden et al., 1996). This statement was tested in a study utilizing two treatment groups: female students who received school-based programs only and students who received both school based programs and mass media interventions. Mass media consisted of television and radio messages. The media targeted group displayed high levels of message appeal and exposure and a 40 percent lower weekly smoking for girls than the school intervention alone. The results indicate mass media interventions that target specific audiences can reduce substance abuse (Worden et al., 1996).

The COMMIT trial (1995) was a four-year multifaceted community-based intervention to help smokers achieve and maintain cessation. The primary group was heavy smokers, yet it was hoped to reach light smokers in the process of the intervention. The trial had no effects on the target group of heavy smokers, a small effect on the light smokers and no effect overall (COMMIT Research Group, 1995).

Most behavioral treatments for smoking cessation are multifaceted. In some cases cessation programs include self-control procedures, stimulus control, and substitute behaviors (Wodarski et al., 1991). Some programs will include stress management and contracting.

There is evidence to suggest that there is a cohort of smokers who are highly addicted and recalcitrant, and are less motivated to quit smoking (Curry et al., 1997; Hughes, 1996). The lower cessation rate among this group is said to be due to an increased withdrawal, long-term craving and the conditioned responses to cues leading to cravings to smoke (Hughes, 1996). Traditional public health and psychosocial programs are unlikely to help this group of individuals; nicotine replacement is shown to have success (Hughes, 1996).

Community Interventions

Many studies have shown that enforcing the legal age of tobacco sales results in reduction of tobacco sales to minors (Forester et al., 1998). In 1996 the Food and Drug Administration issued a restriction on youth access to tobacco products; this included mandatory identification for sale, a ban on tobacco machines and a prohibition against free samples of products. Despite this activity, little is known of the effect of these regulations (Forester et al., 1998). A study by Forester et al. found that community mobilization efforts resulting in policy adoption and restrictions of access to products by youth can affect adolescent smoking rates. Community activities and awareness campaigns in addition to the new policies may have increased the perceptions among students that they would not be able to purchase tobacco. This perception discouraged the students from attempting to buy tobacco products (Forester et al., 1998). The findings of this study are limited in that the results show only short-term effects and the intervention and control groups were made up of only white students. The results do provide a glimmer of hope that policy and community action does make a difference in the quest to put an end to underage tobacco use.

Depression and Smoking

Epidemiological studies have reported an association between smoking and depression (Breslau et al., 1998). People who are depressed are more likely to smoke than people who are not depressed. In addition, smokers who are depressed have a more difficult time quitting (Rabois & Haaga, 1997a). The nature of the link between smoking and depression is still unclear. A study conducted by Rabois and Haaga found that a history of depression is associated with negative coping responses, possibly explaining the link between depression and smoking.

Individuals often use smoking as a coping method for stress; several studies have correlated smoking with anxiety (Wodarski et al., 1991). The coping process may play a very important role in smoking cessation and is beginning to be explored. How individuals appraise their control over stressors and what coping strategies lead to high quit rates have important implications for designing more effective interventions and helping more people quit smoking (Jason & McMahon, 1998). Smokers may be using nicotine to medicate their depressed mood or anxiety. The mood altering effect of the nicotine reinforces the smoking (Breslau et al., 1998).

Researchers have determined that adapted psychotherapies have been useful in treating depression when related to smoking cessation (Rabois & Haaga, 1997a; 1997b). Hall et al. (1994) found that cognitive behavioral therapy was useful in helping smokers who have a history of depression. Yet subsequent research has been unable to replicate this study (Rabois & Haaga, 1997a; 1997b). It has been speculated however that people who are depressed may have a deficit of positive coping skills, triggering the need for smoking. Cognitive behavioral therapy targeted to coping skills rather than depression may be more appropriate treatment for individuals trying to quit smoking (Rabois & Haaga). Smoking interventions that focus on decreasing stress, increasing control, increasing problem-focused coping, and decreasing emotion-focused coping with a social support framework are worthy of further exploration (Jason & McMahon, 1998).

Cost-Effectiveness

The cost of cigarette smoking must be considered on two levels: the cost to the individual and the cost to the public in terms of medical needs, absences from work, and social security.

The dilemma further increases when the profit to the federal government of cigarette sales is factored into the equation. The government makes a profit on tobacco sales and to suggest smoking cessation will decrease this profit.

The average lifetime medical cost of a smoker is estimated to be $6,000 or more than that incurred by a non-smoker (MacKenzie et al., 1994). Research has suggested that because of the lower average lifespan of a smoker, the long-term medical expenditures of smokers may actually equal those of a non-smoker (Barendregt et al., 1997). One study found that non-smokers would incur greater health costs in the long run than smokers.

Three percent of women's and eight percent of men's health expenditures were secondary to the effects of smoking (Barendregt et al., 1997). Approximately $94,700 for women and $72,000 for men are spent on medical expenses during a smoker's lifetime. This is compared with $111,000 for women and $83,000 for men who are non-smokers (Barendregt et al., 1997). Non-smokers live longer than smokers do. The cost-effectiveness of smoking cessation interventions as compared to the medical services needed by an individual who smokes has been well researched (Curry et al., 1998). There is still the tendency for insurance companies to only pay for acute illness (Hughes, 1996).

Chronic Pain

Chronic pain afflicts millions of Americans (NIH Technology Assessment Panel, 1996). The treatment for chronic pain has consisted primarily of drugs and surgery. Chronic pain is a multifaceted experience with physical, emotional, and social consequences (Gagliese & Melzack, 1997). Individuals who suffer from chronic pain often experience insomnia, mood changes, changes in sexual functioning and vocational difficulties (NIH Technology Assessment Panel, 1996).

Pain is the most common complaint leading to visits to the physicians and consequently leads to the spending of billions of dollars in lost activity, wages, and health care costs (Furguson & Ahles, 1998). Assessment is a critical component of the treatment process (Wodarski et al., 1991). This assessment will identify the behaviors that need to be changed and the variables that play a role in the pain behaviors.

Anger is a common emotion experienced by those suffering from pain behaviors (Burns et al., 1998). Researchers believe that individuals suffering from chronic pain often experience resentment and anger about their condition, consequently hindering their ability to benefit from pain programs (Burns et al., 1998). Individuals either express anger or suppress it. Both of these traits are said to be implicated in physical health problems (Burns et al., 1998). Expression of pain could lead to increased back tension and the tendency to express frustration with therapists. Suppressing anger may steer patients from fully exploring their frustrations about their condition (Burns et al., 1998). Anger management techniques may be a necessary component of pain management programs.

Chronic pain is a significant health problem in the United States (Cinciripini & Floreen, 1982; Subramanian & Rose, 1988). Common complaints include such areas as the lower back, neck, head, and face. Social learning pain programs have been largely successful in the management of chronic pain (Cinciripini & Floreen, 1982; Subramanian & Rose, 1988). Keefe (1982) states that if applied early, social learning interventions may be the most effective in reducing chronic pain. However, treatments that are normally used with acute pain are usually ineffective with chronic pain (Keefe, 1982).

Assessment is a key component of the treatment process. Interviews are often used to assess the patterns of pain behaviors and well behaviors (Keefe, 1982). More specifically, the assessment identifies the behaviors that need to be changed and identifies the variables that control the occurrence of these pain behaviors (Keefe et al., 1982; Sanders, 1979). Analysis of this information indicates environmental factors that reinforce the behaviors of the chronic pain sufferer.

Pain behaviors may be influenced by direct reinforcement, avoidance of unpleasant tasks, encouragement of well behavior, and discriminative cues which signal the likelihood of social reinforcement (Cinciripini et al., 1981). Social learning treatment goals for chronic pain sufferers normally revolve around reducing medication usage, increasing physical activity, and reducing interruptions in work and other activities (Cinciripini & Floreen, 1982). Increases in well behaviors also can be achieved through behavioral interventions, but Cinciripini & Floreen state that this occurs more gradually than does the reduction in pain behaviors. Reductions in pain accompany reduction in pain behavior (sighs, moans, limping, spending time in the bed, etc.) and increases in well behaviors will enhance the individual's quality of life by increasing their participation in reinforcing social, recreational, and vocational activities. An excellent two-year follow up study by Subramanian and Rose (1988) indicates the success of cognitive behavioral treatment paradigms.

Treatment Methods

There are many treatment methods used to treat chronic pain, ranging from drug therapy to various alternative methods. The most commonly used alternative methods for chronic pain are outlined below, as well as the efficacy of the various methods.

Hypnosis is an alternative method used in treating chronic pain, often used to induce relaxation (NIH Technology Assessment Panel, 1996). This method has the individual using imagery and distraction. There is a suggestion phase in which the individual is asked to focus on certain goals, such as relieving. There is a also a post suggestion component in which the individual uses the behavior upon termination of hypnosis (NIH, 1996). In a review of studies addressing chronic pain, the National Institute of Health panel (1996), found that data suggest hypnosis is an effective treatment for chronic pain.

Cognitive Behavioral Therapy

Cognitive behavioral therapy is a common method used to help treat individuals suffering from chronic pain (AGS Panel on Chronic Pain, 1998). Cognitive strategies are aimed at altering belief structures, attitudes and thoughts in order to address the pain and suffering (AGS Panel on Chronic Pain, 1998). To be most effective, cognitive therapy should include the teaching of coping skills used alone or in conjunction with pain medications (AGS Panel on Chronic Pain, 1998). Cognitive behavioral therapy can be used alone or in groups, usually requiring between six and fifteen sessions (AGS Panel on Chronic Pain, 1998). In the wake of managed care and the strict guidelines placed on mental health counseling, group sessions are more cost-effective and more likely to be reimbursed by insurance. Keefe et al. (1992) found that when compared to education interventions, cognitive behavioral therapy resulted in lower levels of pain, anxiety, and depression. At the six-months follow-up there was no difference between the groups, though those in the cognitive behavioral group reported lower levels of disability (Gagliese & Melzack, 1997). Cognitive and behavioral techniques greatly influence pain management by their effect on patient attitudes and beliefs regarding treatment. It is obvious that motivation for change and self-control over pain issues affects chronic pain outcomes (Kowal, 2001).

Biofeedback

Biofeedback is often used in conjunction with relaxation (Gagliese & Melzack, 1997). Various studies have outlined the effectiveness of bio-feedback for chronic pain; very few of them include people who are elderly (Gagliese & Melzack, 1997). There has been some evidence that biofeedback and relaxation training do not benefit people who are elderly as they do people who are younger. This difference is said to be because elderly patients have a difficult time learning required response (Gagliese & Melzack, 1997).

Pharmacological Treatments

People who are elderly are more likely to develop adverse reactions to pharmacological treatments for pain. These adverse reactions to drugs often happen at much lower doses than those seen in people who are younger (Gagliese & Melzack, 1997). There adverse reactions may be due in part to changes in metabolism in individuals who are older. Because of these adverse reactions to medications, it is important to consider other forms of treatment.

Headaches

While headaches are a minor health problem in comparison with serious health disorders, their ubiquitous nature makes them of great concern. Chronic recurring headaches afflict 40 percent of the adult population (Ziegler et al., 1977). The principal treatments used with such headaches are various types of both biofeedback and relaxation training which have been proven successful in the treatment of both tension and vascular headaches with 30 percent to 80 percent of patients (Blanchard et al., 1982). This wide range indicates the need for predicting who will respond best to these treatments.

The use of biofeedback in the treatment of tension headaches has become widely accepted. As Lang (1974) and Brenner (1973) point out, however, individuals differ in the ability to benefit from biofeedback. For this reason, more than one type of social learning treatment is often used. Many studies have compared the effectiveness of biofeedback with that of relaxation training and have found them to be equally effective in the treatment of headaches. See Blanchard et al. (1980), Silver & Blanchard (1978), and Blanchard & Andrasik (1982) for reviews of these studies. Blanchard et al. compared the effectiveness of biofeedback and relaxation training on three different types of headaches: tension, migraine, and combined. Relaxation therapy alone produced relief for all three groups with the tension group responding best. Biofeedback produced further reduction in headaches. The overall results were that 52 percent of those with vascular headaches and 73 percent of those with tension headaches were much improved (Blanchard et al., 1982).

It has been hypothesized that reductions in headaches may be mediated by cognitive and behavioral changes which were indirectly created by the biofeedback training (Holroyd & Andrasik, 1982). This hypothesis was supported by data from a three-year study (Andrasik & Holroyd, 1983). A three-year follow up study of tension headache sufferers revealed that improvements achieved by biofeedback treatment can be maintained for an extended period (Andrasik & Holroyd, 1983).

Blanchard et al. (1982) examined the impact of process variables in the social learning treatment of headaches. They examined variables that related to the therapist and variables that related to the patient's practice at home. The variables relating to the therapist (perceived warmth, competency, and helpfulness) were not found to be significant. Variables relating to the regularity of practice at home, however, were shown to be significant. This emphasizes that the primary responsibility for the effectiveness of social learning treatment rests with the person's efforts rather than with the therapist.

Evidence supporting the relationship between headaches and stress has been accumulating in recent years (Holm et al., 1996; Martin et al., 1993). Stress is the most commonly reported precipitant of headaches (Fernandez & Sheffield, 1996; Martin et al., 1993). Establishing a link between stress and headaches raises a number of issues as to why some people suffer from chronic headaches and others do not (Martin et al., 1993). One hypothesis is that the exposure to stressors is different for the two groups. Another possibility is the differences in response to stress. A third possibility is that people who suffer from headaches may be lacking positive coping skills or a strong support system (Martin et al., 1993).

The role of life events is now well documented, and has often shown that the correlation between the frequency of events and subsequent disturbances is of moderate strength (Martin et al., 1993). Life events refer to isolated episodes that provoke significant adjustment difficulties.

These events can range from divorce to retirement. Daily hassles refer to the recurrent irritations associated with day to day living (Fernandez & Sheffield, 1996). In comparing life events with daily hassles, Zarski (1994) found significant but low correlation between life events and headaches. Ivancevich (1986) found that the intensity and frequency of hassles accounted for a significant proportion of the variance. Life events added little to the variance explained. A recent cohort study found significantly higher frequency and average severity of hassles in people with chronic headaches in comparison to the non-headache control group. No significant difference was found between the groups in terms of life events (Martin et al., 1993).

Poor emotional health, particularly depression and anxiety, has been associated with increases in the frequency of headaches (Labbe et al., 1996). Depression is a frequent finding in people with headaches. It is thought that the two are related in a bi-directional manner (Mongini et al., 1996).

Headaches may be a symptom of these disorders. There has been controversy over this issue as to whether chronic headaches lead to depression or anxiety, or whether depression and anxiety lead to headaches. Earlier research thought that depression may cause headaches; current research indicates that depression may be a result of the pain experience (Labbe et al., 1996).

Family history may be a strong determinant of headache activity (Labbe et al., 1996). Family history may represent both genetic and learning influences of headache activity. Makail and von Baeyer (1990) found that children of parents who have headaches were more likely to experience headaches than children of pain-free parents. Children also were found to have significant differences in social skills, delinquency, and general adjustment. This provides evidence for the possible relationship between parents' response to chronic pain and the child's experience of headache (Labbe et al., 1996).

Biofeedback

The use of biofeedback in the treatment of tension headaches has become widely accepted. The efficacy of biofeedback in the treatment of migraines has been well documented (Allen & Shriver, 1998; French et al., 1997). Skin temperature has been shown to be effective. This type of biofeedback is easy for children to learn and is easily incorporated into home-based treatment plans (Allen & Shriver, 1998). Individuals differ in their ability to benefit from biofeedback (Allen & Shriver, 1998; French et al., 1997), this is largely in part because pain is multidimensional and the sensory systems involved are complex (Allen & Shriver, 1998). Generalization involves preparing the patient to carry the learning that may have occurred during the biofeedback session into the real world. The most common method, by far, is a self-control condition which is interspersed between a baseline and a feedback condition (Arena et al., 1997).

Prevention as a Determinant of Health

Sixty billion dollars per year are spent on health care costs and lost work productivity due to heart disease (Paine-Andrews et al., 1997). Most people would agree that prevention of problems of any sort is a good idea. Not only for improved health and quality of life, many agree that a significant reduction in health care costs could be achieved by preventing chronic illness. The role that prevention will play in the light of managed care is unclear (Raines & Erickson, 1997). The standard approach to human services places an emphasis on the deficiencies of individuals (El-Askari et al., 1998). This in turn undermines a client's self-worth in addition to decreasing a sense of responsibility for his or her own well-being. This is an unintended effect of human services programs, but nonetheless a significant one. Literature suggests that there is a strong association between disempowerment and poor health. Therefore, the traditional approach to health programs may be contributing to poor health of individuals, by identifying the problems and attempting to ameliorate them (El-Askari et al., 1989).

The nation's prevention agency the Center for Disease Control and Prevention (CDC) is geared to the prevention of disease, injury and premature death, as well as to promote the quality of life (Speers & Lancaster, 1998). America's metropolitan areas are inundated with a variety of problems that pose serious risks to citizens. Lack of funding, violence, racism, unhealthy behavior patterns and urban stress all add to the increased risk of disease, disability, and premature death (Speers & Lancaster, 1998). The CDC has five objectives: (1) To strengthen public health services; (2) to enhance the ability to respond to urgent health problems; (3) to develop a nationwide prevention program; (4) to promote women's health; (5) to invest in youth.

Smoking prevention programs aimed at teenagers are largely educationally geared (Zittel, 1999). Prevention is particularly important with adolescents because lifestyle behaviors initiated during adolescence become more difficult to change later in life (Pallonen et al., 1998; USDHHS, 1990; Wodarski, 1989). Research has indicated those teens that smoke typically are "light smokers" and have less duration of smoking history, therefore implying that teens have the best probability to utilize behavioral change programs (Pallonen et al., 1998).

Prevention programs should include primary, secondary, and tertiary components (Wodarski, 1989). Preventive interventions are most efficacious when a multidimensional approach is utilized. This approach must incorporate peer influence, family education, schools, and after-school programs (Zittel, 1999).

Prevention programs and educating programs have shown a 20 to 60 percent decrease in cigarette smoking among teens with positive maintenance efficacy for three years following intervention. Research has shown however that positive intervention effects appear to plateau when teens complete high school (Zittel, 1999).

Since 1979 the Oregon Research Group has been dedicated to the reduction of teenage smoking (Lichtenstein et al., 1990). Their main goals include: being able to identify precipitating factors leading to the initiation of cigarette smoking, and the development of habitual, long-term smoking. The Oregon Research Group has also been responsible for the implementation of school based prevention interventions and evaluation of these programs (Lichtenstein et al., 1990). Many studies indicate that most effective prevention programs incorporate interventions, which are sensitive to cultural differences (Botvin et al., 1994; Botvin et al., 1995; Forgey et al., 1997; Moncher et al., 1991).

Implications for Social Work

Much research has been conducted on behavioral treatments that increase wellness. Being a heterogeneous society, more efforts need to be directed at tailoring treatment plans to the individual. The interventions need to meet the client's needs; the clients are not meant to meet the researchers needs (Prochaska, 1996). These plans need to address the individual needs that will in turn increase the probability of adherence and retention to interventions. Social workers need to utilize the treatments outlined above in order to more efficiently work with their clients (Coulter & Hancock, 1989; Berkman et al., 1989; Marshack et al., 1989).

Assessment is critical to the process of behavioral change (Wodarski et al., 1991). The social worker should assess the individual's behaviors that are placing him or her at risk for the development of specific health problems. Methods for reducing or extinguishing these behaviors should be discussed. The social worker should work together with the client to determine a strategy for developing and maintaining a healthy lifestyle. It is important for the social worker to be able to predict whether the individual will be responsive to particular treatment methods.

The best approach is one that employs many interventions that cover all possible variables (Chesler & Barbarin, 1988; Shannon, 1989). The client and social worker must work together in formulating treatment goals. The client must have the bulk of the input, simply because the client is the one who is going to put in most of the effort in achieving change (McClelland, 1989). The assignments given to the client for homework, such as recording, monitoring, counting or rehearsing make the client continually aware of his or her behaviors. Expectation should be explored with confidence that the client can achieve the desired change. It is very important to take small steps, focusing on one behavior at a time, beginning with a simple behavior and then moving on to the more complex behaviors. This step by step process will increase the confidence and build a sense of control.

Specific attention should be focused on cultural factors that are influencing unhealthy behaviors. For example, one of every two black women is overweight. In addition, the prevalence of hypertension and cardiovascular disease among people of African American descent remains a serious health problem (Andersen et al., 1998). Walcott-McQuigg (1995) reported that African American women are less likely to exercise and lose weight and do not feel it necessary to be slim to be attractive. Occupational stress, caregiver issues, racism and sexism are all stressors facing African American women (Walcott-McQuigg, 1995). Simply put, women who are African American may view weight loss and cardiovascular health as the least of their worries. Social workers should assess for these issues before implementing behavioral interventions to increase exercise or facilitate weight loss.

On a more macro level, social workers can help to raise societal awareness about the importance of prevention. This awareness can be raised through in-services at local agencies or hospitals. Social workers can train individuals in stress management techniques, to enhance cardiovascular health. Lobbying for cost-effective signs promoting stair use is a small yet very influential step in exercise promotion.

Social workers should aid in lobbying around anti-smoking campaigns to promote clean air, clean lungs, and a healthy heart. Support for federal bills banning smoking in public areas is very important in promoting wellness. Pressuring local restaurants to offer low fat, healthy foods can do this. Social workers should become involved in programs that promote wellness, such as walk-a-thons and fundraisers.

Women's Health

In terms of research, women have been grossly underrepresented. With the institution of new government agencies placing more focus on women's issues, these gaps are starting to narrow (Edmunds, 1998). More research is needed to address women's issues. In the wake of managed care, there is ample evidence to suggest that members are being denied services. In addition, evidence suggests that utilizing services is becoming more difficult, often with long waiting lists for services (Edmunds, 1998).

New paradigms, methods and measurement tools are needed in order to expand the frontiers of women's health (Harlow et al., 1999). In some areas of research the existing methodology can be adapted in the study of women's health. In other areas, however, new approaches must be made before researchers can understand the etiology of disease (Harlow et al., 1999). In 1997 the Michigan Initiative for Women's Heath hosted a workshop entitled, "Methods and Measures: Emerging Strategies in Women's Health Research" (Harlow et al., p. 139). Three recommendations arose from the workshop: (1) address the bio-psychosocial issues women experience, paying attention to diversity; (2) new methodologies are needed to embrace the richness of women's lives, including an integration of qualitative and quantitative research; (3) interdisciplinary collaboration is appropriate to define and address issues (Harlow et al., 1999).

The treatments and interventions developed by studying one gender can be generalized to women (Blee, 1996). Including both men and women in the same clinical trials is a positive alternative (Blee, 1996). This approach will provide specific information about both women's and men's health. This section contains a critical review of the interventions delineated above.

Risk Factors

There are many risk factors that lead to the declining health of women and the lack of responsibility for their own behavior. This section outlines some specific risk factors leading to the decline of health.

Obesity

Obesity and its associated co-morbid conditions often leads to an impaired quality of life for a large proportion of women, especially those who are African American, regardless of socioeconomic status (Pekkarinen & Mustajoki, 1997; Walcott-McQuigg, 1995). Obesity contributes to the exacerbation of such conditions as osteoarthritis, gallstones, dyslipidemia and musculoskeletal problems in women as well as men.

According to statistics from the third National Health and Nutrition Examination Survey, 32 percent of adults in the United States are overweight. In addition to this, 22.5 percent of adults are obese. Body Mass Index or BMI is the US guideline for classifying weight proportions. The classification for being overweight is having a BMI of 25.0 to 29.9 and obesity as having a BMI of 30.0 or more. Statistics have shown that adults with a BMI greater than 30.0 are more at risk of death (Field, et al., 2001).

In light of increasing health care costs, obesity directly and indirectly contributes to these rising costs. In 1995, health care costs related to overweight and obesity was estimated to be $99 billion dollars. This increased to $117 billion dollars by the year 2000 (Jackson et al., 2002).

Smoking

As mentioned previously, smoking remains the leading cause of premature deaths in the United States (U.S. Department of Health, 1994), accounting for 450,000 deaths per year (Niaura & Abrams, 2002). Approximately 25 percent of people in the United States smoke (Wetter et al., 1998) in spite of the fact that cigarette smoking has been proven to be a major risk factor in heart disease, cancers, atherosclerotic peripheral vascular disease, chronic obstructive pulmonary disease, and stroke. In 1994, 23.1 percent of women and 14.6 percent of pregnant women in the United States smoked (Kendrick & Merritt, 1996). Heart disease is the leading cause of death among women over the age of 34. Twenty percent of heart disease deaths are related to cigarette smoking (Kendrick & Merritt). Smoking is associated with additional hazards for women in their reproductive years (Kendrick & Merritt). Women who smoke and use oral contraceptives increase their risk for cardiovascular disease, as well as increase their risk of infertility, ectopic pregnancy and spontaneous abortion (Wild et al., 1995). The association between smoking and depression emerged from epidemiological studies (Breslau et al., 1998); smoking and affective disorders, especially major depressive disorder, have been linked (Haas et al., 2004). Other studies have shown a strong association between smoking and mood disorders, alcohol and other drug abuse, attention-deficit and hyperactivity disorder and schizophrenia. One study estimated that 41 percent of people with mental illness were smokers. An interesting study showed that among those with a prior history of major depressive disorder many have a relapse of the disorder during efforts of smoking cessation (Niaura & Abrams, 2002). Unfortunately, the nature of this link between smoking and depression remains unclear, but people who are depressed are more likely to smoke than those who are not depressed, and smokers who are depressed have a more difficult time quitting (Rabois & Haaga, 1997a). Smokers have been found to use nicotine as a means of reducing stress and may be using nicotine to medicate their depressed mood or anxiety. The mood altering effect of the nicotine reinforces the smoking (Breslau et al., 1998). During times of stress nicotine is eliminated from the body, and increasing stress results in a faster elimination of nicotine. Therefore, a desire to smoke would follow more often (Todd, 2004).

Research is showing a positive correlation between the issues of body weight and smoking initiation/cessation. This correlation is even more positively related among women. Studies have shown that a person may gain an average of 5 pounds or more upon smoking cessation. Heavier smokers usually have greater weight gain. It is not fully understood how the physiological mechanisms work in this phenomena (Hudmon et al., 1999). It is believed that weight gain is multifaceted. Although an increase in food consumption usually takes place upon smoking cessation, this is not the only factor. Nicotine increases the resting metabolic rate and energy expended. Although significant weight gain is not associated with smoking cessation, many fear the affect of gained weight on their appearance more than the negative impact of smoking on their long-term health (Rigotti, 1999).

Summary

Nearly 70 percent of deaths in the United States are related to preventable illness (Raines & Erickson, 1997). There have been dramatic increases in public health funds. Yet the health of the American public still seems to be deteriorating. Preventive efforts thus far have been of low priority (El-Askari et al., 1998). The CDC has been putting forth effort to focus on the declining health of the American public and has been putting more effort into the prevention of disease, injury, and premature death as well as increasing quality of life. This effort by the CDC will require much effort and cooperation between the federal and state governments (Speers & Lancaster, 1998).

New approaches are important to promote the understanding of the etiology of disease (Harlow et al., 1999). New methodologies are needed which address women's issues and focus special attention toward diverse groups, including an interdisciplinary approach in research. It is not valid to generalize the findings of studies focusing on men to women, and vice versa

(Blee, 1996). The author suggests research on both men and women separately, but also together in the same trials to assess the differences in response to treatment of the two genders.

There are many risk factors that lead to disease. This chapter focuses on three such risk factors: obesity and inactivity, smoking, and hypertension. All of these risk factors can lead to an increase in disease, reduced quality of life and ultimately death. Special attention is given to interventions to ameliorate these risk factors as well as focus on the under-representation of women in research and on traditionally under-served populations.

Traditionally Under-served Populations

Women, in and of themselves, are an under-served population. This section further explores under-served populations including women who are African American, Asian American, and Hispanic American.

African American Women

The overall health of women who are African American is related to their social status within the United States (McNair & Roberts, 1998). African American women have been shown to have lower life expectancies and higher death rates for certain diseases. African Americans have a higher incidence of hypertension (McGrady & Roberts, 1992). One study stated that one out of three African Americans have high blood pressure. Factors related to hypertension include increased age, diabetes, obesity, alcohol use, a high salt diet, a family history of high blood pressure and lack of physical activity (Department of Health & Human Services, 2003a).

After being diagnosed with hypertension, people who are African American have a greater risk of developing organ damage and a higher mortality rate. The mechanisms for this increased risk of organ damage have been linked to an increased sensitivity to norepinephrine while on a high salt diet (McGrady & Roberts). A second mechanism is said to be the psychological effects of stress on people who are African American.

Age adjusted mortality rates in 1992 indicated that the leading causes of death among women who are African American are heart disease, lung cancer, breast cancer, diabetes and AIDS. The differences between heart disease among women who are African American and women who come from a European descent are particularly striking. There are 162.4 deaths among 100,000 for women who are African American, as compared to 98.1 for women who are European American (McNair & Roberts, 1998).

Both infant and maternal mortality rates are higher among women who are African American. The infant mortality rate of babies who are African

American is 2.4 times higher than that of European American babies. The maternal death rate is 3.3 times higher for African American mothers than European American mothers.

There is an inverse relationship between socioeconomic status and health, with lower socioeconomic status being associated with higher rates of morbidity and mortality (McNair & Roberts, 1998). The socioeconomic status of people who are African American tends to be lower than men in the general population. The combination of these two factors makes women who are African American particularly vulnerable to decreased health (McNair & Roberts).

Obesity is a prevalent problem among African American women regardless of socioeconomic status (Walcott-McQuigg, 1995). Fifty percent of African American women in the United States are obese (Department of Health & Human Services, 2003a). African American women are less likely to diet and less likely to perceive themselves as overweight as compared to Caucasian women (Walcott-McQuigg, 1995). Because of cultural factors, some African American women do not feel it necessary to be slim. They do not as often succumb to the societal pressures to be thin. African American women do not share concerns about weight management that Caucasian women generally do. Walcott-McQuigg found that women who are African American experience a variety of stressors that hinder the ability to lose weight, such as, lack of social support, racism, and increased family responsibility. Stressful events have been associated with stress eating behavior, weight gain, and finally obesity. This study, however, consisted of a purposive sample of women who had joined sororities while in college. In addition, women who join sororities are not necessarily representative of the population of college students.

The impact of racism on health is still not understood. There has been little research surrounding the process through which racism influences negative health outcomes (McNair & Roberts, 1998). One hypothesis for the outcomes is that racism reflects the differences between groups resulting from the distribution of resources based on race, leading to the health differences between European Americans and African Americans. Racism also has an adverse impact by limiting access to health care, altering help seeking behaviors, a lower quality of care for people of color, and negative environmental conditions (McNair & Roberts).

A study by McNair and Roberts (1998) states that education is a large step in the reduction of racism among health care professionals. Providers need to be knowledgeable about the socioeconomic factors and the environmental factors as well as the behavioral factors that can attribute to poor health. The authors go on to say that micro level interventions are unlikely to have a significant impact in the case of racism. Instead, they suggest macro level interventions to raise awareness. Public health efforts targeting improved housing and environmental conditions, increased opportunities for employ-ment, health care, and education will all contribute to the quality of life for women who are African American (McNair & Roberts).

Asian American Women

Asian Americans are the fastest growing ethnic group in the United States, with a population of over 3.7 million women in 1990. The term "Asian American" covers over fifty different ethnic groups, speaking over thirty different languages (Helstrom et al., 1998). Though vigorous research on the mental and physical health of Asian Americans began over two decades ago, there is still a lack of empirical information about the health status of this population (Helstrom et al., 1998). For years there has been a prevailing myth that people who are Asian American are very well adjusted. This myth was based on earlier research indicating that Asian Americans have a low divorce rate, high socioeconomic status and high education, and low rate of social deviance. Evidence is now being uncovered that the aforementioned research was an underestimate due to the low numbers of Asian Americans utilizing mental health services (Helstrom, et al., 1998).

Recent research has suggested that women who are Asian American tend to under-utilize mental health and preventative health services, such as breast and gynecological exams (Helstrom et al., 1998). The Department of Health and Human Services reports that Asian Americans have the highest suicide rate for women 65 years or older. One reason may be that it is not socially acceptable in the Asian culture. Shame and guilt are both felt by someone needing mental health services. Additional contributing factors are language barriers of their own or finding services that meet their language needs (Department of Health and Human Services, 2003b).

According to a survey of women at the Asian Health Services in California, 45 percent of Chinese women and 35 percent of Korean women had never had a pap smear. This is consistent with the low survival rate for cervical cancer among women who are Asian American (Helstrom et al., 1998). Vietnamese women are five times as likely to get cervical cancer than Caucasian women (Department of Health and Human Services, 2003b). If caught in its early stages, cervical cancer is "curable." Unfortunately, women who are Asian American typically wait until they have the symptoms, which is too late (Perttula et al., 1999). A study conducted by Perttula, Lowe, and Quon found results similar to the above surveys. The 1987 Cancer Control Supplement questionnaire was translated into Korean and utilized to collect data. The sample consisted of 159 Korean American women. Twenty-six percent of the respondents had never heard of a pap smear and only 34 percent reported having a pap smear for screening purposes.

Women who are Asian American also have a low survival rate for breast cancer. Twenty percent of women surveyed in California who are Chinese, and 43 percent of women who are Korean have never had a clinical breast exam. This is compared to 16 percent of the general population of women in California (Helstrom et al., 1998).

There are several reasons for the under-utilization of health services by women who are Asian American, including language barriers and lack of insurance coverage as well as cultural reasons such as stigma and shame of utilizing mental health and health services. There is a cultural norm among people who are Asian American concerning topics of sexuality. These women are taught at a young age that sexuality is not to be spoken of. This silence may lead to the lack of preventative measures for reproductive health sought by this population.

Jenkins et al. (1999) led a study of the efficacy of a media led education campaign on breast and cervical cancer. Over a 24-month period, a media led community campaign was implemented to promote routine check-ups, clinical breast exams, breast exams and pap tests. The population targeted for this was Vietnamese American women in northern California. To test the impact of the intervention, a pre-intervention telephone interview was conducted with 451 randomly selected women in the intervention area. The same pre-intervention telephone interview was conducted with 482 in the comparison area. Post-tests were completed with 454 women in the intervention area and 422 women in the comparison area. The intervention of the women was to have the tests, yet had no significant effect on being up to date on these preventative tests (Jenkins et al., 1999).

Hispanic American Women

The Hispanic American population is the second largest and one of the fastest growing minority populations in the United States (Woodward, 1998). It is estimated that by the year 2050, one out of four women in the U.S. will be Hispanic American/Latino (Department of Health and Human Services, 2003c). People who are Hispanic American face barriers in access to health care, including insurance coverage. Statistics from the National Center for Health Statistics found that only 71.8 percent of Hispanic people have insurance coverage. In 1994, people who are Hispanic were twice as likely as people who are Caucasian to have no health insurance coverage. The barrier to health care coverage is exacerbated for the one half of those Hispanic women who are heads of households and who are below poverty level (Woodward, 1998). A further study found that there are more Hispanic American women who are uninsured than any other race or ethnic group. This is partly due to most Hispanics being employed by industries that do not offer insurance benefits.

There are also non-financial barriers for women who are Hispanic in terms of obtaining health care, such as language barriers, ethnicity, religion, education, occupation, and culture (Woodward, 1998). Migrant workers who are Hispanic have geographic barriers to obtaining health care. There are typically no health care providers located nearby. According to the National Health Interview Survey data, 93.2 percent of older Hispanic women had not had a mammogram as compared to 83.5 percent of older women who are African American, and 75 percent of women who are Caucasian (Woodward, 1998).

Foreyt et al. (1991) and Kumanyika (1995) stated that obesity is more prevalent among Hispanic women than non-Hispanic, Caucasian women. Williamson (1995) conducted a study that stated Mexican Americans are overweight by 41.5 percent, with 16.7 percent being severely overweight. Comparatively, non-Hispanic, Caucasian women were 24.6 percent overweight and 9.6 percent severely overweight. It is more accepted by Hispanic communities for women to be overweight. It is even considered attractive. A woman considers it a compliment if referred to as gordita buena or pretty little plump one (Johnsen et al., 2002).

Diabetes occurs more often among Hispanic women than among Caucasian women. Almost half of Mexican American women between the ages of 20–74 have borderline high-risk cholesterol levels. It has been discovered that Mexican Americans have a higher rate of heart disease risk and death rates than other American women. This is partly due to a higher rate of diabetes and obesity in this population. Hispanic Americans have the lowest rate of new cancer cases and death rates for all cancer. However, they have higher cancer rates of the stomach, liver and cervix than Caucasians (Department of Health and Human Services, 2003c).

Summary

There is ample evidence to suggest that women of certain minority cultures have an increased risk of certain disease. There are a variety of mechanisms that contribute to these increased risks such as cultural and behavioral factors as well as environmental factors. Women of minority cultures are also less likely to utilize preventive services. This is largely due to barriers in terms of access to health care, both financial and non-financial.

More research is needed that includes women of minority cultures surrounding the prevention of chronic disease. As mentioned above, most research in the past has focused on Caucasian men. Research now needs to include people of minority cultures, with equal inclusion of women in this research.

Research

There are many risk factors that lead to disease. This chapter critically reviews the intervention research for the risk of physical inactivity, obesity, smoking, and hypertension. All of the risk factors lead to an increase in disease, reduced quality of life and ultimately death.

Physical Inactivity

The study of physical activity has proven to be very difficult throughout the years. The two concepts of exercise and physical activity are often confused. If an individual makes a conscious effort to bring up his or her heart rate, this is exercise. Physical activity, on the other hand, is difficult to quantify. Physical activity refers to any bodily movement produced by skeletal muscles.

Research has established the relationship between physical inactivity and chronic health problems. It has been shown that improvement and maintenance of physical activity can reduce "risk of all-cause mortality." It can "improve health and delay death" (Martinson et al., 2001).

Physical activity can improve one's health by reducing risk of heart disease and stroke, high blood pressure, colon cancer, breast cancer, and diabetes, keeping bones, muscles, and joints healthy, reducing anxiety and depression, helping to control weight, controlling joint swelling and pain from arthritis, and increasing energy (Department of Health and Human Services, 2005).

This cause and effect relationship should be of great interest in light of the managed care perspective. Since there is a proven relationship between physical activity and health, it would seem that "health plans and payers may want to invest resources in programs designed to promote physically active lifestyles." Studies have shown that even moderate-intensity physical activity done once or twice per week can greatly reduce the causes of death compared to no physical activity at all (Martinson et al., 2001).

Comparison of Designs

Heirich et al. (1993) conducted a study to determine the effectiveness of four different approaches to reducing specific cardiovascular risks in worksites. One such risk is physical inactivity. The study was a three-year experiment conducted in four automotive manufacturing plants. The four plants were randomly assigned to one of four wellness programs. Each site had base-line data collected. Three years later, a random sample of employees was re-screened. The four interventions were: Site A (n = 493) with the committee offering health education classes to assist in risk reduction, and special events for health awareness were offered. This site was offered an aerobic class, but too few people signed up.

This group became the control group because no exercise program was in operation; Site B (n = 503), a fully equipped fitness facility was established for cardiovascular exercise as well as weight training (Heirich et al., 1993). Athletic trainers were available during all working hours and the fitness facility was well publicized; Site C (n = 481) had two wellness counselors who provided direct outreach and one-on-one counseling for employees who were at high risk. The counselors encouraged employees to develop their own exercise programs. None were offered at this worksite. Counselors were available during 50 percent of working hours; Site D (n = 403) had one-on-one outreach and counseling offered to all employees, as well as organized physical fitness activities during lunch and before and after shifts. The counselors worked about two thirds of working hours (Heirich et al., 1993).

At screening, employees at sites A and C were least likely to exercise with mean exercise levels being significantly lower than those employees at sites B and D. At a three-year follow-up, the worst profile was shown among the employees at site B (the site with the exercise facility), with a mean change of −0.28(p<0.01). Site A, the control group, had a better exercise profile than site B with a mean change of +0.22 (p<0.05). Site C had a mean change of −0.23 (p<0.01). There was no significant change at site B. These results suggest that those sites with one on one outreach were most effective in getting employees with cardiovascular risk to exercise (Heirich et al., 1993).

This study indicates that adding a fitness facility to a worksite does not necessarily increase physical activity among employees. However, the work site containing the facility did not utilize any outreach to the employees. In other words, the mere presence of an exercise facility does nothing to increase physical activity, and in the case of this study, actually may have discouraged employees from exercising. Further study is needed to determine the effect of the fitness facility presence in conjunction with outreach and individual training sessions. The authors do make a case for the effectiveness of counseling in increasing physical activity. There is, however, no mention of what the counseling and outreach entailed.

The authors mention that the sites have similar demographics, though no mention is made as to what these demographics are. The make up of the sample is unknown other than that they are employees of an automotive plant. The lack of information limits the generalizability of the information in the study.

Stages of Change in the Worksite Setting

The Trans-theoretical Model is one of the most recent models used to study physical activity (Peterson & Aldana, 1999). A stage-based exercise intervention in a randomized trial in a worksite setting may help to increase physical activity in individuals (Peterson & Aldana, 1999). The participants in the study are randomly selected employees at a large telecommunication company. Seven hundred and forty-eight employees were randomized into one of the three groups: a stage-based intervention, a generic intervention and a control group. Employees in the stage-based intervention received a two-page written message tailored to their stage of change.

Those employees in the generic group received non-tailored materials based on information taken from the Surgeon General's report on physical activity (Peterson & Aldana, 1999). Six weeks after the materials were received, a follow-up questionnaire was sent to the employees in each of the groups. Sixty seven percent returned the questionnaires resulting in a sample of 527 employees.

To examine the differences before and after the physical activity measures between group differences evaluated using the Duncan follow up, ANOVAs were used. Between-group baseline differences were evaluated using chi-square (Peterson & Aldana, 1999). No differences in terms of demographics were found between the three groups. There were no significant differences in physical activity or stage of change between groups at baseline. At six weeks, the stage-based message group had a 13 percent increase in physical activity; the generic group had a 1 percent increase and the control had an 8 percent decrease (Peterson & Aldana, 1999). The differences were significant between all three groups ($p<0.05$). There were significant differences among the groups in terms of magnitude and direction of stage of change movement. Odds ratios revealed that those in the stage message group were 2.1 times more likely to move at least one stage closer to maintenance as compared to control employees. When comparing the stage group to the generic group, the stage group was 1.6 times more likely to move toward maintenance (Peterson & Aldana, 1999). In short, stage-based messages seem to be more effective than generic messages or no information at all.

In terms of methods and analysis, this study is very detailed and consistent. They do mention the threat of contamination of the study due to the sharing of information by employees, randomized into different groups. The authors further state that with this threat the data show a difference between groups.

As with any study using self-reported data, limitations always exist regardless of the validation of the instrument. Seven days physical activity recall questionnaires have been shown to be moderately accurate in community interventions or interventions with large sample sizes (Taylor et al., 1984). The sample of this study was largely female (60.4 percent), Caucasian (83.5 percent), well educated (85.7 percent), with some college and young (79.3 percent) under age 45, limiting the generalizability of the study.

Self-help Physical Activity Interventions

One problem encountered by worksite exercise promotion programs is that they tend to attract people who are already physically active, or highly motivated to make a lifestyle change (Marcus et al., 1998). Marcus and colleagues conducted a study to "enhance motivational readiness for the adoption of physical activity" (Marcus et al., p. 249). Eleven worksites that were already participating in the Working Healthy Research Trial were participating in this ancillary study called "Jump Start to Health."

The sample of this study consisted of 1559 employees at eleven different worksites that were individually randomized to one of the two treatment conditions (Marcus et al., 1998). The average number of employees at each worksite was 200. The interventions consisted of either a tailored motivational self-help activity intervention or standard physical activity habits. The same data were collected at three-month follow-ups.

At follow-up the participants were divided into two groups, completers (903) and non-completers (656). The two groups differed significantly from each other in terms of marital relationships.

The authors state two significant limitations to COMMIT interventions. The first being that the protocol for the intervention may have limited some communities from undertaking additional activities that may have had significant impact on smoking cessation.

The second limitation is the lack of emphasis placed on macro level changes (environmental and policy changes) that may have been powerful in terms of smoking cessation (COMMIT Research Group, 1995).

Smoking

Depression and Smoking

As cited by Haas et al. (2004), there is a positive link between smoking and affective disorders, particularly major depressive disorder. Research states that mood may be a definitive factor in smoking behaviors (Haas et al., 2004). As cited by Todd (2004), studies have demonstrated a positive link between stress and cigarette smoking. The demands of work and other social stressors are also linked to the desire to smoke. It is shown that women are more likely to smoke during stressful times.

The explanation of the relationship between smoking and depression is in the use of smoking as self-medication because of the mood altering characteristics of nicotine (Breslau et al., 1998). Breslau et al. utilized data from a five-year epidemiological study of 1007 young adults. The incidence and odds ratios are based on prospective data. The results revealed that a history of major depression at baseline increased the risk for progression to daily smoking with an odd ratio of 3.0 and confidence interval of 1.1–8.2. The results further indicated that a history of daily smoking at baseline significantly increased the risk of major depression with an odd ratio of 19 and a confidence interval of 1.1–3.4. The hypothesis that major depression decreased the potential of smoking cessation was not supported (Breslau et al.).

The generalizibility is also limited due to the age range or there may be separate causal mechanisms that lead from depression to the progression to smoking and smoking to depression.

It is a plausible explanation that individuals who are depressed may self medicate. It is more difficult to explain the reason for the influence of smoking on depression. Some findings state that smoking may affect neuro-transmitters. More research is needed to further explain the possible link (Breslau et al., 1998).

Depression, Smoking and Coping

There is a possibility that formerly depressed smokers are lacking in cognitive coping skills. Rabois and Haaga (1997b) examined the relationship between depression and smoking.

According to the authors, if you take smoking away from people who are depressed, you may be removing an effective mood-regulating coping skill. Participants were recruited by poster and newspaper ads in Washington, DC. A one hundred-dollar prize drawing was offered for participants. The sample consisted of 87 individuals. Eighteen smokers had a history of depression, 23 smokers with no history of depression, 21 non-smokers with history of depression and 25 smokers with no history of depression. Depression was defined as having experienced five out of nine of the DSM-III-R for major depressive episode for at least two weeks (Rabois & Haaga, 1997b). Smokers were defined as individuals who reported smoking at least 10 cigarettes per day for at least three months. Ex-smokers were excluded.

The measure included a demographic and smoking questionnaire, The Ways of Responding (WOR), to serve as a measure of cognitive coping. The WOR is said to have good inter-rater agreement for coding. The validity of the WOR was supported in that the WOR coding and subjective quality judgments correlated positively with a measure of learned resourcefulness. Psychology students were trained to rate the WOR responses for the study (Rabois & Haaga, 1997b).

Smokers with a history of depression did not differ significantly in current depressive symptoms from non-depressed smokers. Smokers with a history of depression did significantly exceed non-depressed smokers in past depressive symptom severity (Rabois & Haaga, 1997b). Both groups of depression and both groups of non-depressive symptoms did not differ significantly from each other. A two-way ANOVA on depression history multiplied by smoking status on WOR positive scores yielded non-significant main effects for depression history and smoking status. A parallel two way ANOVA on WOR negative scores revealed no main effect for smoking status and no interaction between smoking status and history of depression (Rabois & Haaga, 1997b).

In short, a history of depression, regardless of smoking status, is associated with negative coping skills. This finding may help to explain the link between a history of depression and the failure to quit smoking. The study further indicates that people with a history of depression tend to lack positive coping skills and may benefit from incorporation of cognitive behavioral therapy principles in smoking cessation programs (Rabois & Haaga, 1997b).

The authors delineate some limitations to the study. One such limitation is that even though secondary analysis indicated that the differences between groups were not influencing the main results of the study, it would probably be better if the groups were matched more closely on age and sex (Rabois & Haaga, 1997b). A second limitation is that the history of depression groups and the non-depressed groups obviously differed in current depressive symptoms, especially among non-smokers. These differences may result in the misattribution of depression vulnerability and correlates of current depression. A third limitation mentioned by the authors is that depression was measured by self-report, introducing some bias. In futures studies, it may be wise to utilize structured interview to assess depression.

A limitation not mentioned by the authors is the lack of representation of minorities. The sample was made up of 77 percent people who are white, while only 10 percent were African American, five percent Asian American and the other five percent were of other nationalities. In addition to this, the authors do not mention where the posters for recruitment were placed. There is no way to determine if socioeconomic status is representative, though the authors do mention that the sample is highly educated, leading to the assumption that the sample is from a mid to high income.

Smoking Cessation

Family Physician Brief Intervention

Physicians are often trained in smoking cessation techniques. Richmond, Mendelsohn and Kehoe (1998) studied whether or not physicians utilized these techniques. The authors aim to determine the utilization of brief smoking cessation interventions six months after attending a training workshop and to examine the effect of reinforcement contact on physician utilization.

One hundred ninety-eight physicians attended a workshop to be trained in smoking cessation techniques. The physicians were then randomized into one of two groups: the contact group (n = 98), which received reinforcement contact from the workshop trainer and a second group, the non-contact group (n = 100) who received no additional reinforcement. The sample size yielded an effect size of 0.30 or greater at an 80 percent power. This also took into account a 25 percent loss to follow up (Richmond et al., 1998). Doctors in the contact group received three brief telephone calls at two weeks, two months, and four months after the training workshops. Ninety-six of the physicians received three phone calls. Two of the physicians were away for the holidays. The calls were designed to encourage continued use of the program. Physicians in the no contact group had no further follow-up.

At a six-month follow-up, 88 percent of the physicians in the contact group and 84 percent of the no contact groups were users of smoking cessation literature ($p = 0.06$). Full time physicians in the contact group were distributing more booklets than the no contact group ($p = 0.05$). Sixteen to 20 percent of the patients were abstinent from smoking. This study is the first to measure long-term utilization of smoking cessation interventions by family physicians. This is also the first study to demonstrate the effect of brief reinforcement contact by phone (Richmond et al., 1998).

Smoking Cessation for Hospital Patients

Hospitalization offers an opportune time to initiate smoking cessation behaviors. First, most hospitals ban smoking. Second, an illness often motivates smoking cessation (Rigotti et al., 1997). Third, patients are somewhat of a captive audience. Rigotti et al. tested to determine whether the hospital is an appropriate opportunity to initiate smoking cessation. The authors developed an intervention to test the efficacy of a brief, bedside smoking cessation-counseling program in a randomized controlled trial at a hospital in Boston, MA. The intervention consisted of a 15-minute bedside counseling session, written self help materials, chart prompts reminding physicians to advise smoking cessation, and up to three weekly counseling phone calls after discharge.

In any study, retention of the participants is a significant issue. The authors of this study anticipated that 15 percent of the participants would be unavailable for follow-up. The sample consisted of 650 individuals, which allows for an 80 percent power to detect a 10 percent group difference.

The effectiveness of the intervention was determined by comparing the outcome measures between the groups using intent to treat analysis. The people who were unavailable for follow up were counted as smokers. No significant differences in socio-demographics were found at baseline except for age. The control group was slightly older than the intervention group (Rigotti et al., 1997). Groups did not differ in terms of medical history, reason for admission, surgical procedure, or length of stay. There were no differences found in beliefs about smoking-related health problems, smoking behaviors, quality of life, or alcohol consumption.

All patients lived until hospital discharge. Fifteen patients died before a one-month follow-up; thirty-five died before a six-month follow-up and were excluded (Rigotti et al., 1997). The intervention and control groups did not differ in terms of mortality rate at one-month or six-month follow-up. At a one-month follow-up, the intervention group maintained abstinence at a higher rate than the control group. The cessation rates were statistically significant for one-month abstinence. At a six-month follow-up, the differences between groups had narrowed: 17.3 percent of the intervention and 14 percent of the controls reported not smoking in the previous week (p = 0.26). Sustained abstinence since discharge was reported at 13.7 percent of the intervention patients and 10.1 percent for the controls (Rigotti et al., 1997).

When using self-report measures, there is always the issue of over- or under-reporting of information. To validate the self-report of non-smoking at six-month follow-up, saliva samples were requested from the 85 percent of the self-reported non-smokers still living in Massachusetts. Non-smoking was confirmed in only 54 percent of the self-reported non-smokers. Confirmation rates did not differ significantly between interventions and controls. The main reason for non-confirmation was refusal of saliva testing (Rigotti et al., 1997). For those who provided a saliva sample, non-smoking was confirmed in 80 percent.

Few studies have tested the effect of smoking cessation in hospital inpatient care regardless of reason for admission. Rigotti et al. (1997) have illustrated this type of intervention is cost-effective and short term. The statistical analyses of the study are very thorough and take into account a variety of biopsychosocial issues. The attempt to obtain saliva sample allows for the securing of more reliable data about abstinence. This study does have its limitations. The physicians administering advice were not trained in how to give this advice. The advice given is likely to affect the smoking cessation patterns of the intervention group. In addition, people who do not own telephones were not included in the study, which may lead to problems in generalizability in terms of socioeconomic status. This study is also not generalizable in terms of ethnicity. The intervention group in this study was 90 percent Caucasian, with the control group being 94 percent Caucasian. The authors do not address these limitations.

Gender and Smoking Cessation

Gender differences often exist in response to brief interventions (Whitlock et al., 1997). Some studies have indicated that women are more likely to cut back on smoking rather than quitting. A study by Whitlock et al. explored whether gender differences exist in response to brief intervention. Researchers utilized the results of a study conducted in 1988. The sample size of this study was 2707, all of whom received physician advice before being randomized into one of four treatment groups, one of which was the physician advice-only control group. Whitlock et al. aimed to determine whether gender affected the results of this study.

The gender comparisons of baseline characteristics, clinic participation, and smoking outcomes were analyzed by a two-tailed continuity adjusted chi-squared analysis or t-tests. Gender comparisons were also made on smoking-related and health-related attitudes in ongoing smokers by the same tests. Movement in stage of change and relapse was analyzed by two-tailed Mantel hazel chi-square analyses (Whitlock et al., 1997). Minorities were equally represented among both male and female smokers. Females were less likely to be married, to have post high school education or be employed as a professional. Females were also less likely to report trying to change their dietary habits. Women have a lower Body Mass Index than men and consider themselves to be overweight. In terms of health, women were more likely to have acute respiratory disease documented. More men than women had a history of smoking related cardiovascular disease recorded within the past five years. Female smokers had an average of 4.7 clinic visits as opposed to 2.9 clinic visits for men (Whitlock et al., 1997).

This study is interesting in that it assesses the differences between males and females by conventional methods and by incorporating the Trans-theoretical Model, which is based on the stages of change and a participant's readiness to change. This study, like many others, does not adequately represent people of color, with only 7.1 percent of women being of color and only 8.5 percent of men being of color. This lack of minority representation compromises the generalizability to people who are not Caucasian. In addition, the participants are all members of an HMO. Participants who are members of an HMO are either employed in an organization or are in a financial situation that allows taking out an individual insurance plan. The use of only individuals with health insurance compromises the generalizability of the results to individuals of a lower socioeconomic status or those in a service profession that does not offer health insurance.

Hypertension

Bio-Behavioral Treatments

Both biology and behavior play a role in the development and control of hypertension. Fahrion et al. (1986) conducted a study on the effects of bio-behavioral treatment for essential hypertension. The sample consisted of 77 patients diagnosed with essential hypertension. The sample was comprised of twenty-nine women and forty-eight men with a mean average age of 48 years. Some of the participants were on hypertension medications, while others were not. The baseline data was collected through self-reported blood pressure readings over the course of one week from the participants' home readings.

The interventions was multifaceted, including biofeedback training for hand and foot temperature to achieve vasodilatation, cognitive explanation of the rationale for biofeedback training, diaphragmatic breathing exercises, relaxation techniques, home practice of self-regulation and home monitoring of temperatures (Fahrion et al., 1986). The participants were trained in psycho-physiologic control in the clinic for one hour per week. The outcome measures were the achievement of muscular relaxation, to breathe diaphragmatically and to become normotensive (blood pressure of no more than 140/90). Treatment continued until the patient achieved all of the training goals, stabilized over time, or dropped out of the intervention (Fahrion et al., 1986). A categorical analysis was conducted based on the criterion of treatment success with hypertension (Fahrion et al., 1986). Of the fifty-four participants who were taking medication for hypertension, 58 percent were able to discontinue the medication in addition to lowering their blood pressure by 15/10mm Hg. Nineteen of the participants who were taking medications were able to cut the dose in half in addition to lowering their blood pressure by 18/10mm Hg. The remaining four participants taking medication showed no improvement (Fahrion et al., 1986). The participants who were not taking the medication showed similar results.

A repeated measure ANOVA was performed to examine changes in the four separate groups of participants; the medicated patients with follow-up information, the medicated patients with no follow-up information, the un-medicated patients with follow-up information, and the un-medicated patients with no follow-up information. There were significant reductions in systolic blood pressure for the medicated patients with follow-up information with an F of 25.95 and a p of <0.001, the medicated patients with no follow-up information with an F of 14.60, and a $p < 0.005$, the un-medicated patients with follow-up information with an F of 6.51 and $p < 0.005$, and with the un-medicated patients with an F of 37.52 with $p < 0.01$. Similar resultss were found with diastolic blood pressure (Fahrion et al., 1986).

This study does have its limitations, the first of which is that there was no control group, making it impossible to determine that the changes were due to the intervention or to outside effects or a regression to the mean (Fahrion et al., 1986). The baseline for the study was short, only one week. A longer baseline may present a more accurate picture of blood pressure. The authors also mention that there may be a discrepancy between how the participants are supposed to take their medication and how they actually do take it. A limitation that the authors do not mention is the lack of sufficient minority representation with only three participants being of minority status. This compromises the generalizibility of the results of the study.

Behavioral Stepped Treatment

Glasgow et al. (1989) hypothesized that stepped care in the form of self-monitoring, biofeedback, and relaxation in a stepped program can complement anti-hypertensive medications in lowering blood pressure, with the ultimate goal of less medication resulting in an avoidance of side affects. The study sample consisted of fifty-one patients whose blood pressure was medically controlled and received usual care. The participants were recruited at an HMO clinic serving a largely blue-collar population.

Participants were matched in groups on the basis of medication requirements (diuretics, beta-blockers alone or with diuretics, vasodilators alone or with one of the aforementioned medications). The intervention lasted one, four or seven months, depending on response to treatment, with a follow-up of 12 months. The control group protocol lasted for 19 months (Glasgow et al., 1989). The sequence of monitoring, then biofeedback, and then self-monitoring was chosen because an earlier study showed this sequence to be effective. Each participant was given his or her own sphygmomanometer to facilitate self-monitoring of blood pressure. A baseline blood pressure was collected for one month prior to the intervention.

Medication requirements for the intervention group declined to levels significantly lower than those of the control group with a $p < 0.05$. This was true throughout the follow-up phase for all the different drug groups combined. When the drug groups were analyzed separately however, only those patients taking diuretics and/or beta-blockers showed a decrease in the need for medication (Glasgow et al., 1989). The authors state that the blood pressure levels did not change when the levels of medication were adjusted, indicating that the stepped care in conjunction with medications can be complementary. The authors further mention that the stepped care intervention is easily reproducible and in this case was shown to be effective in comparison to usual care. This study does have its limitations. The study had a very high dropout rate during the baseline phase. Of the possible 506 participants, 211 were disqualified due to pre-existing medical conditions (Glasgow et al., 1989). One hundred eleven participants declined to volunteer. Of 167 participants who signed the release form, sixty-one patients withdrew during follow up, leaving 102 patients. Many perspective participants ($n = 90$) expressed a general lack of interest in the study. The authors make no mention of the script followed during the recruitment phase. This is important information to know so as to avoid similar dropout patterns in the future. In addition, the authors make no mention of any retention activities utilized during the study. These activities may have prevented some of the dropout activity.

Interestingly, there were more than twice as many Caucasian people in the study than people who are African American. African Americans have a higher incidence of hypertension and a higher mortality rate from the disease than do Caucasians (McGrady & Roberts, 1992).

Summary

This section provided a critical analysis of the interventions mentioned in the previous chapters by delineating the specific interventions used to treat inactivity and obesity, hypertension, and smoking.

The research surrounding physical activity typically involved randomized controlled trials utilizing t-tests, chi-square tests to determine differences between groups and ANOVAs to determine the significance of these differences. Worksite interventions as a whole were deemed to be ineffective.

In terms of smoking, the research suggests a link between smoking and depression (Breslau et al., 1998; Rabois & Haaga, 1997a). The research surrounding cessations suggests that women and men are equally likely to utilize smoking cessation programs. The research further suggests that smoking cessation programs need not be expensive. Simple suggestions from a physician may not in and of themselves result in smoking cessation, yet may implant the importance of quitting.

The information addressing hypertension suggests that behavioral treatment for hypertension may not lower blood pressure enough to avoid medication. The research does suggest that behavioral treatment in conjunction with hypertensive medication will help to reduce the need for high doses of hypertensive medications.

One significant limitation of many of the studies was that they did not adequately represent people of minority cultures; this was evident of most studies regardless of the topic. Further research is needed with adequate representation of minority cultures as well as adequate representation of individuals of lower socioeconomic status.

8 Prevention

Cost Saving for Reducing Health Care Costs

Prevention strategies are often successful in reducing physical illness. Can they also help alleviate mental illness? These two areas are intertwined. Effective health care cannot treat one area independently of the other. A focus on community studies, multiple risk factors, and cost efficiency can lead to effective prevention interventions. Empirically based models for preventive care strategies already exist. They demonstrate cost-effectiveness in delivering health care (APA, 2006; Chamberlin, 2005; Greer 2005; Stambor, 2006).

The current publicly funded family planning system provides contraceptive services for about 4.5 million women, mostly high risk. Without these services, there would be an estimated 1.2 million additional unintended pregnancies and 500,000 additional births each year (Forrest & Singh, 1990). Infant mortality rates would surely increase. The Allen Guttmacher Institute reports that federal and state governments spend approximately $400 million annually for contraceptive services, but they save approximately $1.8 billion on services to those women who would otherwise give birth. This demonstrates the cost-effectiveness of prevention and early intervention programs.

Unfortunately, deficit-ridden state and local governments are cutting back prevention programs in an attempt to balance their budgets. This is certainly not cost-effective. One informative example of this policy is the curtailing of family planning services and teen pregnancy programs. Savings in public medical costs alone are estimated to be $4.40 for each $1 spent on contraceptive services for the typical clinic patient (Forrest & Singh, 1990). Savings in income support and social services are even greater.

Almost 10 million women of reproductive age have no health insurance. Over 5 million such women are insured under plans that do not provide maternity coverage, primarily for financial reasons (U.S. GAO, 1990). These women represent a potential budget buster for federal and state governments. They have the highest incidence of low birthweight babies, are more likely to use publicly funded family planning services, and tend to have far more unwanted pregnancies (NCHS, 1990). State insurance commissioners should pressure insurance companies to provide family planning services for teens, single, and poor women.

Emotional problems and mental disorders represent a substantial cost to society, though the public grossly underestimates them. The effect of mental disorders on our families, work, and society are often hidden. Few are aware that more people die from suicide than from homicide in the United States (U.S. Bureau of the Census, 1994; Kersting, 2005a).

Depression afflicts 17 percent of American adults (Kessler et al., 1994) and can produce dysfunction as great or greater than that of a chronic physical illness (Wells et al., 1989). According to the Surgeon General's (1999) report on mental health, 20 percent of children and adolescents experience symptoms of a mental disorder during the course of a year and 75–80 percent of those fail to receive appropriate treatment (cited in Weissberg et al., 2003). Mood disorders contribute to some of the major causes of death such as smoking and drinking (McGinnis & Foege, 1993; Schoenborn & Horn, 1993). Even health care providers may overlook mental illness in their patients (Depression Guideline Panel, 1993).

Mental disorders place an extraordinary financial burden on the country, in addition to their cost in human suffering and lost opportunity. The 1990 economic cost of mental disorders, excluding alcohol abuse, was estimated at $98 billion. The cost of drug abuse was estimated at an additional $66 billion. Despite these enormous expenditures, only 10 percent to 30 percent of individuals in need are estimated to receive appropriate treatment.

History

Since the founding of the National Association for Mental Health by Clifford Beers in 1909, groups have periodically called for an increase in promotion of mental health and the prevention of disorder. The mental health establishment's typical response has been benign neglect. Exciting advances in prevention are developing during this time of public impatience with societal and psychiatric problems (Heller, 1996).

Heller (1996) writes early advocates of prevention were long on rhetoric and short on empirical data. Moralistic claims were frequently presented as reasoned policy. For example, in the late nineteenth century, a eugenics perspective prevailed advocating sterilization of the developmentally delayed and mentally ill, forced confinement in institutions, and immigration quotas to prevent pollution of the gene pool. President John F. Kennedy used prevention rhetoric in his 1963 message to Congress proposing establishment of federally funded community mental health centers. Goals for reducing the incidences of new cases (primary prevention) or the duration and severity of symptoms (secondary prevention) were spoken without any indication of how to implement them.

The historical mandate of physical and psychiatric medicine is to restore sick bodies and minds. Established treatment protocol focuses on treating complex disorders suffered by individuals. The last two decades have revealed the financial and social costs of a high technology health system primarily treating disease. While individual cases benefit from treatment, this benefit is not reflected in a decrease in the incidence of new cases of disease and mental disorders. Social problems fester as the mental health profession focuses on treating individuals (Heller, 1996).

Emergence of Prevention Science

The National Institute of Mental Health (NIMH) formed the Center for Prevention Research (CPR) in 1982 to consolidate and coordinate government sponsored prevention research. Though there were prior individual efforts in mental health prevention science, CPR and its sponsored research centers dramatically increased support for controlled prevention trials. CPR's later incarnation, the Prevention Research Branch within NIMH, had a two-fold mission, testing atheortical intervention strategies and collecting empirical evidence about theoretical causal models of change processes (Heller, 1996).

Prevention science was coined at the 1991 NIMH sponsored National Prevention Conference to describe a research discipline primarily focused on the systematic study of precursors of dysfunction (risk factors) and health (protective factors). Reciprocal interplay between basic risk factor research and controlled intervention trials was envisioned. Basic risk and protective factor research informs the design of prevention intervention; and field trials of preventions yield insights into factors contributing to risk vulnerability or resistance. The relationship between the presence of risk and protective factors and observed incidence of disorder was believed to be complex with disorders linked with multiple risk factors and each risk factor linked with multiple disorders (Heller, 1996).

Cost Analysis

In addition to understanding the effectiveness of preventive care in reducing health risks, it is also essential to note the importance of utilizing a cost analysis for any services provided. Cost–benefit analysis can be used to determine the cost efficiency of preventive care. This analysis has gained increased attention as an important aspect of program evaluation. Even before the recent series of economic recessions, there was increasing pressure on social work administrators to be accountable. Gross (1980) describes the two elements of accountability as "the need for social workers to exhibit that what they do is effective, i.e., that social workers are able to achieve socially valued goals, and that these goals are realized efficiently, i.e., in the cheapest way possible" (p. 31).

Federal cutbacks in funds for social services and shifting responsibility for many programs to the states have agency administrators increasingly concerned with costs in beginning new programs, maintaining existing program levels, or retaining any funding at all for some programs. Administrators need information related to program costs as well as program outcomes in order to compete successfully for scarce resources. They also need this information in order to make hard decisions about internal programming, that is which programs to retain and which to terminate or modify. Cost–benefit analysis, adapted from the field of business and economics, has been cited as useful in facilitating such decision making (Levin, 1983).

Cost–benefit analysis is essential to understanding the cost efficiency of a program. This analysis is a process through which program costs and effects (benefits) are identified and quantified. Both costs and benefits are expressed in dollar amounts and then compared. If benefits exceed costs, assuming no limitation of funds, the program is considered worthy of funding. If a limitation exists, a cost–benefit analysis can be used to establish funding priorities. Stokey and Zeckhauser (1978) state the fundamental rule of cost–benefit criteria is, "in any choice situation, select the alternative that produces the greatest net benefit" (p. 137). Thus, cost–benefit analysis is concerned with maximizing gain from marginal output.

Cost-effective analysis differs from cost–benefit analysis in that it requires a monetary value to be assigned to program costs but not to program benefits. The assumption is that program objectives are based on society's desire to achieve certain goals. Thus, decisions are focused on choosing the program that will meet the already identified objective in the most efficient way.

Cost-effective analysis cannot help establish program priorities. It can help find the most efficient way of obtaining priorities established by some other means (Buxbaum, 1981). Benefits are specified in some non-monetary units, that is, number of foster care children returned to their biological families. Cost-effective analysis determines how many units of benefits are associated with alternative approaches to reaching the same objective.

Social agencies face ongoing problems evaluating service effectiveness. Criteria for assessment of service effectiveness are difficult to establish. Such criteria are often tied to theories of human behavior that are either explicitly or implicitly used as a rationale for various intervention programs. Many of these theories have yet to be systematically evaluated in regard to practice effectiveness.

Perhaps one criterion that can be used universally is the extent to which utilization of a specific theory and its practice implications produces desired outcomes in client behaviors (Fischer, 1971, 1978; Wodarski & Feldman, 1973). However, even when such a criterion can be specified, problems of measurement arise.

Efforts have been made to develop measures to assess client outcomes in relation to service provision (i.e., Hudson, 1982). While many practitioners are using these and similar measures on an individual basis with clients, few agencies have instituted such procedures as a means of evaluating overall agency effectiveness. Agency effectiveness, as measured by outcomes of service provision, will require continuing attention and additional research. Without such documentation, it will be difficult for administrators to justify high cost programs or services in times of resource scarcity.

Increasing emphasis on agency evaluation will necessitate that schools of social work develop curricula that will address multiple aspects of agency assessment. Evaluation skills must be taught which will enable future graduates to develop and implement various types of assessments. Continuing education and in-service training programs can be organized to develop these competencies in social workers already in practice.

The comprehensive agency evaluation must encompass many perspectives and foci. It must also utilize data from various sources, including consumers, workers, and community service providers, in addition to accounting departments. The agency that engages in these multifaceted assessments can develop a holistic view of overall agency functioning, which identifies both areas of weakness and of strength.

From a cost standpoint, the interventions that the social service systems have chosen are extremely costly and highly unproductive for both client and practitioner. The literature indicates that services should be structured in a short-term manner. For an MSSW beginning social worker earning $33,000 direct salary and (0.32) fringe benefits equaling $10,560, 32 hours of intervention would cost $348. Thus, the possible savings realized through prevention are obvious.

Prevention: A Paradigm

Prevention strategies should include training in areas such as (a) relaxation, (b) assertiveness, (c) self esteem, (d) anger management, (e) stress management, (f) problem solving, (g) urge control, (h) parenting, and (i) employment skills. Training in these areas can be used as a base for preventing a multitude of potential physical and mental health problems. Each of these skills can be developed through education and support networks. These skills are crucial elements of preventive care.

Relaxation can be learned through systematic techniques through which the client can alternate between tensing and relaxing muscle groups. This will not only aid clients physiologically, but will also help them to identify by body signals those situations which are anxiety and anger provoking (Bernstein & Borkovec, 1973). Clients should be trained in progressive muscle relaxation to reduce the effects of stress. Proper breathing for relaxation, guided imagery, and methods of monitoring the effectiveness of the relaxation are tools taught to clients to aid their relaxation training.

Altering client dissatisfaction about interpersonal relationships and the perception of themselves as lacking in social skills is important in preventing stress and violence. Clients must learn how to interact with others in meaningful and satisfying ways. Facets of a program developed by Lange and Jakubowski (1976) involving conversational skills training, use of appropriate nonverbal communication, and development of assertive behavior are recommended to decrease stress from inadequately met social needs.

Cognitive anger control is another skill useful in preventing physical and mental health problems. Clients learn to identify stresses that can provoke anger and subsequent violent behavior. They develop cognitive relaxation skills to reduce the effects of stress. Obtaining the skill of cognitive anger control necessitates learning how to receive assertive statements, and to deal with the anger of others. Finally, clients must develop appropriate communication, assertiveness skills, and practice alternative behavior such as stimulus removal, in anger provoking situations (Wodarski & Wodarski, 1998).

Stress management is another important aspect in prevention training. Clients learning these skills first learn to isolate antecedents and triggers of stress. Clients need to understand or learn behavioral reaction cues that call for certain behaviors. After learning to recognize possible triggers of stress, clients need to be able to recall the steps to stress reduction. Finally, clients need to evaluate the outcomes of their stress management.

Clients who have difficulty coping with the daily problems of living should be taught a problem solving approach based on the work of D'Zurilla and Goldfried (1971), Spivack, Platt, and Shure (1976) and Schinke and Gilchrist (1984). Problem solving skills involve (a) learning to orient oneself to the reality that problems occur, being able to handle them, and overcoming the tendency to react on impulse or do nothing (b) defining the problem in operational terms and formulating its different aspects, (c) brainstorming to generate possible solutions, (d) choosing a solution based on the expected consequences pro and con, and (e) evaluating the process as new information is gained through implementing your choice. These skills involve clients isolating and defining a behavior to be changed, using stimulus control techniques to influence rates of problem solving behavior, and using appropriate consequences to increase or decrease a behavior.

The basic principles of social learning theory should be taught to clients to enable them to manage situations involving drugs. Social learning theorists emphasize that drug abuse is learned from the consequences of drug use. These consequences most often include stress reduction, removal from an unpleasant situation, or an excuse for otherwise unacceptable behavior. In order to teach clients to control urges to use drugs and alcohol, clients must first be taught the signs and symptoms of alcohol abuse, how to identify specific drug urges, and triggers for substance abuse.

Clients need to learn new methods for relaxation and managing stressful situations. They need to develop feeling, talking, and listening skills. Soon, clients must begin to learn (a) nonverbal communication, (b) expression of negative feelings, (c) social skills, and (d) initiating conversation. Eventually, clients need to learn (a) the social skills of giving and receiving complements, (b) the assertiveness skills of making requests, (c) drink and request refusal, and (d) to develop an awareness of anger management.

In the final stages, clients learn problem solving techniques, how to manage negative thinking and to cope with urges to use substances. Finally, clients learn relapse prevention in the form of (a) self-monitoring, (b) recognition of warning signs, (c) planning for emergencies, and (d) having fun without alcohol or other drugs.

Parenting skills can also be useful in preventing physical and mental health problems for the parent and the child. Teaching parents the components of child management can help develop parenting skills. First, teach parents the behaviors that are appropriate for children at different developmental stages. For example, parents may be taught the initial language skills of children, their ability to identify objects or to carry out requests. Parents must also learn how rewards and punishments (e.g., verbal praise, eye contact, or verbal reprimands) can control behavior. Parents need to learn how to isolate and define a behavior they want changed (e.g., throwing objects or increasing sibling interaction). The parents then learn the use of appropriate consequences to either increase or decrease a behavior.

Stimulus control techniques can also be taught to parents. They will influence rates of behavior. For example, parents could restructure physical aspects of the home, or change their voice level, eye contact, or facial expressions. Simple graphs and tables could then be used to chart behavioral change to evaluate intervention effectiveness.

Lack of employment or the ability to gain employment can lead to mental and physical health problems. These problems stem from obvious financial, as well as self-worth issues. Employment skills can be taught to clients in three sections. First, using group discussions that focus on using a motivational influence throughout the job-seeking process. Second, using exercises to help clients obtain a job, including (a) role playing the interview experience, (b) planning out appointments, (c) learning conversation skills, (d) how to dress appropriately, (e) how to market their skills, and (f) how to present their strong points in an interview. Lastly, teaching problem solving skills.

The rationale for the job program is well documented in the literature. Specifically, data indicate that employment interventions reduce the recidivism of crime involvement by increasing the possibility of leading a law-abiding life (Glaser, 1994). Exercises and videotapes are used to help participants apply the tools they have learned and help in skill maintenance. Group process utilizes peers as resources and generates an environment that can effectively promote the learning of job acquisition skills.

Community Preventive Strategies

Universal strategies for the prevention of physical illness, such as the Stanford Three City Study and the follow up Five City Study (Farquhar et al., 1990), have effectively used intensive media campaigns aimed at cardiovascular risk factors. Universal strategies such as these are possible when they are relatively inexpensive, acceptable to the host community, and likely to reach and influence those at risk (Kellam & Rebok, 1992; Chamberlin, 2006).

Comparable studies using public community institutions have been used to reduce the risk for mental disorders. For example, in Baltimore, first grade classrooms provide an opportunity to build academic mastery through sophisticated changes in curriculum and teaching methods that reduce aggressive behavior through sustained use of cooperative activities.

Strategies targeting interventions at persons at risk for mental disorders have been explored for promoting both physical and mental health. The crucial advance is to recognize the link between targeted and universal strategies. In the Stanford health studies, persons at high risk for heart disorders were recruited for more intensive individualized health training. Likewise, in the Baltimore study, children with difficulties were recruited for more intensive interventions.

Community as an Arena for Prevention

The National Institute of Mental Health (NIMH) (1995) report noted the importance of careful community studies. First, the characteristics of communities may determine the trajectories of development and the timing of critical developmental transitions. Generalizations from preventive trials are most secure when they are applied to communities similar to the study community. The report also noted the importance of understanding community dynamics that may influence the acceptance of any form of professionally based interventions and community characteristics influencing retention of effective interventions as part of community routines.

The report noted the importance of community studies in determining variations, within and across communities that may influence the prevalence of mental disorders and the major risk factors for them. For example, community economic conditions influence hospitalization rates for mental disorders as well as risks for suicide. In particular, the report was concerned that preventive intervention research involve culturally diverse populations and take into account multiple risk factors within those communities.

Many promising prevention programs now under development target multiple risk factors such as (a) poverty, (b) job loss, (c) discrimination, (d) caregiver burden, (e) medical problems, (f) divorce, (g) lack of social support, (h) school failure, and (i) family conflict. These programs will provide an important base for more rigorous research trials with larger and more diverse samples.

Preventive services need to be offered in settings other than mental health centers, particularly in schools. They should sometimes focus on problems that transcend the usual definitions of mental disorders. In this way, preventive services will open up opportunities for the application of psychological and other behavioral approaches across a broad range of areas.

Although the National Academy of Sciences' Institute of Medicine (IOM) report focused specifically on prevention research, clinical preventive services are already being provided on a routine basis, particularly in the primary care system (Mrazek & Haggerty, 1994). Clinical preventive services include immunizations, screening tests and counseling intervention for problems such as smoking (Gold et al., 1993). However, a focus on mental health prevention services has generally been absent.

Risk Factors

Studies that estimate attributable risk factors for mental disorders are beginning to appear (Bruce, Takeuchi & Leaf, 1991; Dryman & Eaton, 1991). Biological and psychosocial risk and protective factors for the onset of depression are (a) having a parent or other close biological relative with a mood disorder, (b) a severe stressor, (c) low self-esteem, and (d) having a low sense of self-efficacy. Being female and living in poverty are also risk factors for depression.

The IOM report emphasizes that risk and protective factors are often common to many disorders; it is important to understand their interaction. Risk factors should always be viewed in relation to their prevalence in the normal population. Reducing specific risk factors, especially at crucial times in the development process, may be more beneficial than attempting to reduce risk factors in general (Mrazek & Haggerty, 1994).

However, it is important to note that a focus on risk and protective factors as precursors to dysfunction should not exclude a focus on social injustice and the epidemiological evidence linking poverty and social class to rates of mental disorders. One problem with using public health interventions to prevent mental illness is that many mental disorders are socially acquired maladjustments. Stress from poverty, physical and sexual abuse of children, child neglect, isolation, exploitation, low self esteem associated with involuntary unemployment, low social status, and discrimination on the basis of race, gender, and sexual orientation result in socially disapproved behaviors we label mental illness.

Prevention should not be approached piecemeal with a focus only on individual risk factors, but through a political campaign that squarely confronts discrimination and social inequity (Perry & Albee, 1994). Landsman (1994) states the ecological embeddedness of behavior cannot be overlooked if any type of preventive measures is to be truly effective.

Attributable Risk

It is important, when dealing with the science of prevention, to understand attributable risk. This is the maximum proportion of cases that would be prevented if an intervention were 100 percent effective in eliminating the risk factor. For example, even though smoking is a major risk factor for lung cancer, eradicating smoking completely would not completely eliminate lung cancer. The proportion of cases that would be prevented represents the attributable risk due to smoking (Mrazek & Haggerty, 1994). This concept highlights the limits on incidence reduction that even powerful interventions can be expected to produce.

Social Action

Perry and Albee (1994) agreed that effective prevention would require societal change and political action to achieve equal rights and to reduce the stresses of *discrimination* and *exploitation*. Heller responded "articulating a moral position without evidence of intervention effectiveness is not enough, because an equally compelling morality for many persons is one that champions individual initiative and responsibility as the primary ingredients needed to overcome social adversity" (p. 1124). This statement harkens back to a time when many Americans embraced the romanticized Horatio Alger myth that anyone could pull themselves up by their bootstraps. Because we now have more knowledge of the effects of structural obstacles and their effects on individuals and groups than we did a half-century ago, this myth is no longer credible.

Life Skills Training Intervention Model

One model that can be used in creating prevention strategies based on skills training is the Life Skills Training Intervention Model (LSTIM). Data surrounding the use of the LSTIM, in addition to the uses of the Teams-Games-Tournaments (TGT) teaching method, provide rational and empirical support for the development of prevention and health education programs for clients. This model has rationale and elements in common with other preventive approaches based on a public health orientation (Caplan, 1964) which are variously called grabbed pre-exposure (Epstein, 1976), immunization (Henderson et al. 1972), psychological inoculation (Meichenbaum, 1975). Here the intervention goal is skill building to strengthen clients' resistance to harmful influences in advance of their impact. Three components comprise this preventive model: health education, skills training, and practice applying skills in troublesome situations (Wodarski & Wodarski, 1993).

Clients need accurate information to make informed health choices. Simply exposing clients to facts about unhealthy consequences of certain behavior is painfully inadequate. Past health education programs made poor judgments in assuming exposure to training materials guarantees learning. Information only programs have had few long lasting effects (Haggerty, 1977; Marsiglio & Mott, 1986). Accurate perception, comprehension, and storage of new information is a complex process that depends on individual receptivity and the nature of the information presented (Mahoney, 1974). Perceptual errors, selectively ignoring, misreading, or mishearing certain facts and selectively forgetting information can create discrepancies between facts presented and facts received and remembered. LSTIM addresses this potential problem by asking clients to periodically summarize presented concepts in written and verbal quizzes. Correct responses are then reinforced; errors are detected and clarified. Furthermore, peers are used as teachers, thus enhancing a commitment to healthy behaviors.

Another critical issue overlooked in traditional health education programs is helping clients relate specific facts and observable risks to themselves and to their own lives. Relational thinking is the process by which abstract information becomes part of one's everyday reality (Mahoney, 1974). This relational process is best accomplished by actively involving clients in gathering and assimilating information. Examples of this include special information collecting assignments (e.g., interviewing resources, conducting surveys) and experimental exercises requiring verbalization of facts of choices in personal terms (e.g., each time I have sex and don't use birth control, I risk pregnancy). Direct discussions of illusions and faulty thinking patterns used to conveniently ignore important health facts (i.e., it can't happen to me; I can quit anytime I want to; I never have an orgasm, so I don't have to worry about getting pregnant), also aid the personalization or relational process.

However, even personalized information is of little value if clients lack the skills to use it. Translating health information into everyday decision making and behavior involves cognitive and behavioral skills. LSTIM thus emphasizes skills for making effective short- and long-term decisions and assertive and communication skills needed to implement decisions.

Cognitive skills training is adapted from research on problem solving (D'Zurilla & Goldfried, 1971; Spivack et al., 1976). Problem behavior is associated with peer norms and expectations. Realistic decisions about how to act must, therefore, consider responses of significant others. The ability to anticipate both interpersonal and health consequences of behavior, generate alternative action strategies, and arrive at the best choice is crucial to health promoting decision making. An example is training focused on sexual behavior.

Following discussion of birth control advantages and disadvantages, adolescents anticipate possible difficulties using this information in social situations such as not knowing whether or when to initiate discussion, handling personal embarrassment, and dealing with partner reactions. Adolescents generate several possible plans specifying when, where, and how the discussion could occur. They predict the probable outcomes of each plan and select the one most feasible (Wodarski & Wodarski, 1993).

Training also focuses on behavioral skills necessary to transform decisions into action. Based on established assertiveness and communication skills training procedures (Lange & Jakubowski, 1976; Schinke et al., 1979; Schinke & Rose, 1976), training presents verbal and nonverbal aspects of good communication to help clients learn to (a) initiate difficult transactions, (b) practice self disclosure of positive and negative feelings, (c) refuse unreasonable demands, (d) request changes in another's behavior, (e) ask others for relevant feedback, and (f) negotiate mutually acceptable solutions.

The final and most important phase of the LSTIM involves the client practicing the application of skills in a variety of potentially risky interpersonal situations. Extended role-playing interactions provide clients with opportunities to recall and make use of health information, decision-making techniques, and communication skills. In role-playing, clients practice responding to increasingly insistent demands, receive feedback instructions and praise to enhance their performance.

Practice applying skills also takes the form of homework assignments involving written contracts to perform certain tasks outside the training environment (e.g., initiating discussion of birth control with a dating partner). Clients also practice skills for dealing with social pressure. For example, clients might practice specific situations where individuals apply pressure to persuade others to consume excessive amounts of drugs. Clients would practice reactions in this scenario, to statements like: one drink won't hurt you; what kind of friend are you?; just have a little one, I'll make sure you won't have any more.

Clients are also taught components of appropriate reactions, such as (1) to look directly at the pusher when responding, (2) to speak in a firm, strong tone with appropriate facial expression and body language, (3) to offer an alternative suggestion such as I don't care for a beer, but I'd love a Coke, (4) to request that the pushers refrain from continued persuasion, and (5) to change the subject by introducing a different topic of conversation.

The Teams Games Tournaments Model

The Teams Games Tournaments (TGT) technique, developed through two decades of research at the John Hopkins University Center for Social Organization of Schools, is an innovative, small group teaching technique. Though the method was created for school students, it serves as an example for other small group settings and populations. This method is grounded in current theory and applies to diverse problems, populations and settings. TGT provides clear criteria for evaluating program effects. The technique gives each client an equal opportunity to achieve and to receive positive reinforcement from peers by capitalizing on team cooperation, the popularity of games, and the spirit of competitive tournaments. Group reward structures set up a learning situation wherein the performance of each group member furthers the overall goals of the group (Wodarski et al., 2004).

Adolescents: a Prototype

The skills training intervention and TGT models can be effectively used as tools of prevention in dealing with adolescent issues such as sexuality, substance abuse, and so forth. Adolescents need to be equipped with specific knowledge to deal with potential peer influences on cognitive and social behaviors.

The skills training approach may be thought of as overt (verbal and nonverbal components of overt social behaviors) and covert (internal skills affecting cognitive, self-control and problem-solving abilities across all social settings and circumstances) learned behaviors that maximize chances for obtaining positive reinforcement from social interactions while minimizing cost to self and others (Gilchrist, 1981). Social skills training typically consists of the following components: (1) a rationale as to why a given social behavior is desirable, (2) an opportunity to observe examples of the behavior (i.e., modeling), (3) an opportunity to practice the behavior, usually in role-play situations, and (4) corrective feedback regarding performance (Rusch, 1986).

Research indicates that it is necessary for adolescents to (a) successfully develop relevant educational competencies; (b) handle current problems and stresses; (c) anticipate and prevent future problems, and (d) advance their mental health, social functioning, and economic welfare. Initially, adolescents' social skills attitudes should be assessed. Subsequently, adolescents should participate in a series of psycho-educational courses, including vocational enrichment (Azrin, 1978), enhancing interpersonal relationships (Lange & Jakubowski, 1976), managing stress and building social responsibility (Schinke & Gilchrist, 1984), determining alternatives to aggression and dealing with feelings (Goldstein et al., 1980), and problem solving (D'Zurilla & Goldfried, 1971; Spivak and Shure, 1974).

A variety of psycho-educational methods are employed in skills training, including (a) individual and group counseling, (b) self-assessments, (c) live and videotape demonstrations, (d) development of self-efficacy, (e) behavioral rehearsal with counselor, (f) peer reinforcement, (g) individual and group contracts, (h) buddy systems, and (i) progress logs. Most of these therapeutic strategies are delivered through a group work approach (Feldman & Wodarski, 1975; Wodarski, 1981).

Even though recent years have witnessed a growing emphasis on group treatment, relatively few youths at risk are treated in this manner. The provision of service in groups offers youths interactional situations that more frequently typify many of their daily interactions. Services that facilitate the development of behaviors that enable people to interact in groups are likely to better prepare adolescents for participation in larger society. It will help them learn the social skills necessary to secure reinforcement (Feldman & Wodarski, 1975; Wodarski, 1981). Social learning theory posits that if a behavior is learned in a group context, it is likely to come under the control of a greater number of discriminative stimuli. Therefore, greater generalization of the behavior can occur for a broader variety of interactional contexts.

The group of the various skills programs is intended to capitalize on the adolescent's dependence on peers. Group identity and cohesion should be fostered within groups of adolescents. Group support can be mobilized to aid individuals at moments of particular difficulty (Ross & Glaser, 1973) and it provides a context where new behaviors can be tested in a realistic atmosphere (Feldman & Wodarski, 1975). Adolescents can get immediate peer feedback and support regarding their problem solving behaviors and they are provided with role models to facilitate the acquisition of requisite social behavior (Meyer & Smith, 1977; Rose, 1977; Wodarski, 1981).

Lack of interpersonal relationship skills often contributes significantly to an adolescent's inability to attain and maintain educational success and to their general dissatisfaction with life. Services structured in a group manner should help these individuals practice necessary social skills to facilitate their acquisition, thus enhancing their interpersonal relationships and educational opportunities. Additionally, adolescents may feel emptiness, social isolation, and a sense of failure . . . and should benefit from the support derived from the group (Wodarski & Bagarozzi, 1979).

The use of small learning groups over the last fifteen years has been applied to many classroom problems; the teaching of verbal reading, arithmetic, health skills, and discipline. The Teams-Games-Tournaments (TGT) technique was developed through extensive research on games as teaching devices, on small groups as classroom work units, and on task and reward structures used in the traditional classroom. The TGT technique has a successful history with subjects that traditionally have been hard to teach, such as nutrition and social studies. The TGT model fully utilizes a reward structure that emphasizes group rather than individual achievement (Feldman & Wodarski, 1975; Wodarski et al., 1980).

Group instruction is preferable to individual classroom instruction because the group learning situation most closely resembles the setting in which adolescents make their decisions regarding high-risk behaviors. High-risk behaviors most often take place in group settings; knowledge acquired in group settings is more likely to be used when in similar peer settings than knowledge acquired through individual, separate means (Allman et al., 1972; Feldman & Wodarski, 1975; Wodarski & Bagarozzi, 1979). From the perspective of the educator, the group method allows for a broader range of learning experience. Students have the opportunity to learn while interacting with peers in a friendly, exciting game.

The three basic elements in the TGT technique, which promote motivation and interest in learning, are teams, games, and tournaments. When TGT is used, all students have an equal opportunity to succeed because all students compete against members of other teams who are at similar achievement levels. Therefore, the points earned by low achievers are as valuable to the overall team score as the points earned by high achievers.

Before beginning the education phase of the program, students are assessed for their level of high-risk behavior knowledge. The completion of the pretest of knowledge provides the basis for division of students in four member teams. The teams are organized into high achievers (those with a high level of knowledge about high-risk behaviors), middle achievers (those with moderate levels), and low achievers (those most lacking in knowledge). Team composition is heterogeneous, with one high achiever, two middle achievers, and one low achiever on each team. The average achievement level is approximately equal across teams. The team remains intact throughout the period when TGT is used. The day before a tournament, team members hold a practice session to study together or to fill out worksheets reviewing the material covered that week. Peer tutoring is encouraged.

The students compete against members of other teams on instructional games composed of short answer questions designed to assess and reinforce the material taught in class. Students play these games in weekly tournaments. Each student is assigned to a tournament table to compete individually against two other students. Each of these three students represents a different team. The students at each table are of comparable achievement levels. Points are earned for each game question answered correctly and at the end of the tournament, the top, middle, and low scorers get a fixed number of points. In addition, each player receives certain points for participating in the tournament. The points a student earns are used to determine whether he/she will stay at the same level table. This process encourages students who have increased their achievement levels to keep working. The points are added to those earned by other members of the student team to compute a team score. The individual and team scores should be ranked and publicized in a tournament newsletter for the class.

The education units centering on high-risk behaviors can be presented for 50 minutes each day for four to seven weeks. The first three days of each week are to be devoted to learning concepts regarding high-risk behaviors through exercises, discussions, and various participatory activities. The fourth day should be focused on working in the TGT teams on worksheets in preparation for the tournament, which is to be held on the fifth day of each week.

Incorporating this model into a preventive strategy will not only successfully aid in the prevention of health and mental problems, it will be possible to do so in non-traditional settings. Incorporation of this model and others like it will provide care providers with the tools necessary to effectively help communities while also increasing efficiency.

Research

Botvin (2004) states a growing number high quality studies demonstrating the effectiveness of some prevention approaches with particular problems. The push is on to identify and disseminate the most effective prevention programs. Ringwalt et al. report current estimates suggest fewer than 30 percent of American schools are implementing evidence-based programs (cited in Botvin, 2004).

The poor fidelity common in the field may explain poorer than expected performance of programs taken to scale. Potential barriers in school settings include a lack of training and support, limited resources, classroom over-crowding, disciplinary problems, teacher burnout, and multiple competing demands. Fidelity sometimes competes with the perceived need for adaptation. Improved fit may increase buy-in, perceived relevance, and extend utilization of the program (Kersting, 2005b).

Castro et al. (2004) state fidelity and adaptation are both important aspects of prevention programs. Universal (culturally blind) programs will fail to prompt community participation and this may skew outcome effects. Conversely, a culturally appealing program lacking validation is of unknown therapeutic value. Some form of adaptation is pervasive in communities across the country. Community-based program design will often combine a top-down (social planning) and a bottom-up (grass roots) approach. The primary goal is to develop a culturally equivalent version of a prevention model.

Backer (2004) recently proposed a set of program adaptation guidelines that emphasizes balancing fidelity and adaptation (cited in Castro et al., 2004). Finding the Balance is a dynamic 12 step approach. Cultural adaptations must move beyond the surface and address core values and beliefs. Dimensions guiding adaptation include cognitive information processing (e.g. language, age), affective-motivational (e.g. gender, ethnic background), and environmental (e.g. ecological aspects). Two basic forms of adaptation involve modifying content and modifying form of program delivery.

The Society for Prevention Research (SPR) strategic plan is (1) promote federal and state initiatives on integration of research and practice, (2) develop standards for level of rigor required for confident conclusions about efficacy of practices, and (3) develop and promote use of data systems to measure trends in positive youth development and influential state and local factors. Emphasis is shifted from efficacy research to effectiveness in real world settings.

Conclusion

Despite the statistics about the number of people who have been seen and helped by mental health services, most people eventually come to understand that increased treatment activity does not reduce the incidence of new cases of disorder. Although individual patients might benefit, in the long run, society as a whole is not better off as a result of this large investment. Thus the implementation of an empirical based preventive approach is long past due.

Prevention strategies, often successful in reducing physical illness, can also help reduce mental illness. Mental illnesses, such as depression, can be as debilitating as chronic, physical illness. Empirically based models already exist that demonstrate the cost-effectiveness of prevention in health care delivery. Still, debt-ridden state and local governments are cutting funding for prevention programs such as family planning clinics.

The Prevention Paradigm focuses on training in relaxation, assertiveness, self-esteem, anger management, stress management, problem solving, urge control, parenting and employment skill. This can be provided through education and support networks.

Community Prevention Strategies can combine universal and targeted programs. Universal programs, such as the Stanford Three City and Five City Study, effectively used an intensive media campaign targeting cardiovascular risk factors. This type of strategy is possible when it is relatively inexpensive, acceptable to the host community and likely to reach and influence those at risk. The Baltimore study gave a more intense, targeted intervention to first graders who did not respond to the universal intervention. It has been suggested that a lack of effectiveness of the universal strategy can be used as an indication of the need for a more targeted intervention.

The Positive Youth Development Project (1996) found several interventions effective in reducing problem behaviors such as drug and alcohol use, aggression, truancy, smoking, and high-risk sexual behaviors. These interventions promoted bonding, social, emotional, cognitive, behavioral, and moral competencies; fostered resilience, self-determination, spirituality, a clear and positive identity, belief in a future, pro-social norms (healthy behaviors), and offered the opportunity to practice and receive recognition for pro-social behaviors.

Many prevention research programs have similar methodological complications; (a) difficulty in adhering to a strict randomized, controlled trial design, (b) high attrition of participants, (c) lack of documentation of fidelity in delivering the intervention, (d) lack of multiple measures of outcomes from multiple sources and (e) insufficient long-term follow-up, which can prevent the collection of outcome data on incidence of multiple disorders. In addition, there is wide variability regarding whether a program with positive outcomes will go on to field trials or be adopted as a service program. Issues of dissemination must clearly be addressed. Conversely, service programs can provide good leads regarding intervention and would profit from being experimentally validated.

The IOM report concluded there is no evidence preventive interventions can reduce the incidence of mental disorders at this time. However, examples exist indicating risk factors associated with the onset of disorders can be reduced, as can subclinical symptom levels. Research in prevention has been hampered by lack of funds. Long-term studies are necessary to prove the efficacy of prevention (Mrazek & Haggerty, 1994). For example, whether early preschool education contributes to a more productive, less criminal citizenry took 20 years to prove (Heller, 1996).

Biological and psychosocial risk factors for some mental illnesses have been identified. For example, risk factors for depression are (a) having a parent or close biological relative with a mood disorder, (b) a severe stressor, (c) low self-esteem, (d) low sense of self-efficacy, (e) being female, and (f) living in poverty. Risk factors and protective factors are often common to many disorders. It is important to understand their interaction and the prevalence of the risk factor in the general population. This focus on risk and prevention factors should not overlook the issue of social justice or epidemiological evidence linking poverty and social class with rates of mental illness.

Summary*

Emerging Trends

Evaluation of Practice

More investment will be placed in the future on practice intervention with clients. Practitioners will continue to combine research skills in developing practice technology in conceptual advancement in the understanding of human behavior. Standards of practice will be developed. Data systems will facilitate the execution of research pertinent to the practitioner's needs that are being developed by agencies. More sophisticated questions will be posited. There will be a move from polemic questions, such as "is casework effective?" to "what technique, and worker and client intervention, treatment contexts, duration, and relapse prevention procedures interact to produce the greatest client change?" The main questions will be: "were the services offered the client instrumental in a change for the better and if the alternatives exist what costs will be evaluated to access which interventions cost the least?" (Breckler, 2005; DeAngelis, 2005; Kersting, 2003; Wodarski, 2000).

Components of successful treatment packages will be analyzed (Levant 2005). In task-centered casework (Dziegielewski et al., 2005; Paul, 1969), essential aspects of the model that elicit specific client behaviors will be identified, such as structure, expectations, enhancing commitment procedures, planning task implementation, analyzing obstacles, modeling, rehearsal, guiding practice, and summarizing. The aspects will provide data for answering six complex questions of a practice technology.

Reid (1992) suggested that the task-centered model became mainstream in the late 1960s with psychosocial and problem-solving casework. When comparing task-centered case management to behavioral approaches, it encompasses a broad range of issues to include a client's relationship to diverse environmental systems.

Reid (1992) states that task-centered case management offers intervention approaches which complement common problems encountered by social

---

*   Chapter written with the assistance of: Carla Kimble.

workers. Task-centered case management can resolve problems which may stem from difficulties sustained by families and children, depression, alcohol abuse, inadequate resources, and psychosocial difficulties combined with mental and physical illness.

Research should help resolve critical legal dilemmas regarding practice that plague the profession at this time. If left unresolved by the profession, it will be up to the courts to set guidelines. For instance, what are the traditional acceptable standards for practice? What is adequate treatment and where should it be provided? What qualities should the change agent possess? How long should treatment be provided? What happens if there is no change in the client? (Bernstein, 1978; Johnson, 1975a, 1975b, 1975c; Wodarski, 1976).

Moreover, if accumulated data attest to the efficacy of particular treatment approaches, those treatment technologies that restrict the client's civil liberties the least and demonstrate superior effectiveness over the other approaches will have to be utilized (Thyer & Wodarski, 2007). Under the legal doctrines of equal protection and least restrictive environment, all individuals are constitutionally entitled to the same privileges or social services. Thus, if two or more technologies achieve the same results, the technology that restricts the client's liberties the least, in such terms of personal resources as money, time, and energy, must be used. Judges have placed their rulings concerning treatment issues on these two criteria (Martin, 1974, 1975; Wodarski, 1976).

Role of Research in Education

The role of research in social work education will increase dramatically at all degree levels within initial training in the relevance of research in social work at the baccalaureate level (Baer & Federico, 1978). The curricula will include courses based on empirical knowledge, the practice techniques derived from a verifiable empirical base, and the relevant practice issues that can be resolved through research. More faculty will engage in research relevant to practice and will move to knowledge development with applications. Moreover, student and beginning practitioners will begin to integrate research findings substantially into practice.

Stein (2003: 62) states that

> The readiness to break new ground, and to be exposed to new ideas, has been manifested most particularly in United States social work's reform tradition, at the turn of the century, during the depression of the 1930s, and in its recent resurgence. This spirit of inquiry is also evident in the research efforts of social work in the United States, in the growing emphasis on research teaching in its professional schools, and in increasing alertness to relevant developments in allied fields of knowledge.

As discussed above, new variables must be isolated and new types of theories must be developed to alter the factorial complexity of human behavior effectively. Another development will be the incorporation not only of task-centered casework theory in social work practice, but of empirically based theories of human behavior and behavior change: on accurate empathetic understanding, nonpossessive warmth, genuineness (Parloff et al., 1978; Truax & Carkhuff, 1967). Many graduate programs in social work will incorporate into their curricula theories of interpersonal attraction, attribution, and relationship formation; game theory and discussion theory; effect of organization on behavior; nonverbal communication; and matrix therapy.

Future research will likely unravel the complex relationship between societal experiences and human behaviors. For example, an issue which will be addressed in the future but which the field has virtually ignored is how to construct a society using macro-level interventions versus individual interventions to prevent or facilitate certain pro-social behavior (i.e., more emphasis will be placed on preventive service if it is cost effective).

In the past, employment opportunities for social workers in criminal justice, health, marriage and family counseling, and human services were uncontested. Now social workers must compete with colleagues in non-traditional human services programs using empirical theories. The curricula of social work schools must, therefore, incorporate knowledge bases of social psychology that will provide an empirical base for practice techniques (Dziegielewski et al., 2005: 7).

> Stein (2003) affirms that the initial reason in teaching social work in agency practice was on understanding individual behavior, and dealing with individuals, casework had a long "head start." Some courses in schools dealt with a broad spectrum of social problems, only a few schools began with improving social welfare services as their main objective. Social work education in the United States formed an advantage with the close relationship and the need for daily practice, and the application of imagination and academic study to the pursuit of more systematic and effective social work method, based on education.

Rapid Assessment Techniques

Accurate assessment of client, worker and agency attributes for effective practice will become the norm (Wodarski, 1981a, 1981b, 1985; Thyer & Wodarski, 2007). Fortunately, there are accurate assessments of clients available to professionals (Streever et al., 1984). The majority of professionals also operate under the false practice assumption that all depressed clients are homogeneous in nature rather than heterogeneous (i.e. that 100 depressed clients need the same treatment, whereas interventions are more effective when tailored to each client).

The goal of social work education is to equip the practitioner with the fundamental tools necessary for accurate assessment, an essential element of effective intervention at all levels of social work practice, whether it be individual, group, organizational, or societal level. Rigorous assessment in training is considered to be a *sine qua non* for qualitative training and social work practice. No matter what powerful techniques the change agents possess, insufficient time spent on assessment results in ineffective or irrelevant intervention because an accurate evaluation of the client's difficulties has not occurred.

The assessment process is prevalent in obtaining information surrounding your client. Toseland & Rivas (2005) state that the assessment process narrows as data is collected, organized, and decisions are made regarding how to intervene, how to cope with an issue or how to remedy the problem.

In the last decade, a number of rapid assessment scales have been developed to facilitate obtaining information necessary for workers to make adequate assessment of their clients (Rittner & Wodarski, 1995; see Chapter 3). The measurement instruments and procedures, designed to provide ongoing feedback, and to assess and to document client change during the helping process will be incorporated in social work education.

Prevention

Lochman (2001) found the following:

> The process of identifying new preventive interventions should not only be permeable and responsive to current changes in preventive intervention approaches and technology, it should also continually refine and test existing interventions.

Social work will stress prevention interventions (Wodarski & Wodarski, 1993). The helping professions have a history of dealing with individuals only after they have exhibited behavior problems. To resolve this deficiency, the social work profession should facilitate thorough research on the preventive and educative roles that can be assumed by social workers, and criteria should be developed for early intervention.

Prototypes of this approach may be found in courses of parental effectiveness, sex education, and marital enrichment. Parental effectiveness courses should focus on helping parents develop better communication and consistent child management skills, two variables that research has shown are necessary conditions for successful child rearing (Hoffman, 1977). Likewise, sex education and marital enrichment programs should prepare young adults for the requisites of marriage with effective communication skills, problem-solving strategies, and conflict resolution procedures (Collins, 1971; Ely et al., 1973; Lederer & Jackson, 1968; Rappaport & Harrell, 1972; Satir, 1967).

In another example, adolescents identified as high risk for poor coping with daily life can be taught a problem-solving approach based on the works of D'Zurilla and Goldfried (1971), Goldfried and Goldfried (1975), and Spivack and Shure (1974). The general components emphasized are:

1   How to generate information
2   How to generate possible solutions
3   How to evaluate possible courses of action
4   How to choose and implement strategies through the following procedures:

    (a) General introduction on how the provision of certain consequences as stimuli can control problem solving behavior
    (b) Isolation and definition of a behavior to be changed
    (c) Use of stimulus-control techniques to influence rates of problem-solving behavior
    (d) Use of appropriate consequence either to increase or to decrease behavior

5   How to verify the outcome of the chosen courses action

Family Intervention

Data indicate that parents whose adolescents are at risk face multiple social and psychological difficulties. The clearest finding about adolescents at risk is the lack of knowledge by the parent or parents and the consequent lack of effectiveness in managing the child's behavior in a manner that facilitates his or her psychological and social development. It has also been pointed out that another common feature of relationships between parents and adolescents at risk is unrealistic expectations by the parents on what is appropriate behavior of their child (Cowen & Work, 1988; Howing et al., 1986; Kersting, 2003; Patterson & Forgatch, 1987; Wodarski & Thyer, 1989).

Another empirical finding of note has been in the high degree of strain evident in families. Family interventions patterns have been characterized as primarily negative; that is, parents engage in excessive amounts of criticism, threats, negative statements, physical punishment, and a corresponding lack of positive physical contact, and so forth (Bock & English, 1973; Brandon & Folk, 1977; Brennan et al., 1978; Hildebrand, 1968; Robin & Foster, 1989; Robinson, 1978; Suddick, 1973; Vanderloo, 1977). In review of this finding, a comprehensive prevention approach should include appropriate interventions that teach family members about the problems adolescents face, health issues, substance-use issues, communication skills, problem solving, and conflict resolution.

Greenberg et al. (2001) reported that

> Interest in prevention is also reflected in the goals that have been set for our nation's health. One of the original objectives of Healthy People 2000

was to reduce the prevalence of mental health disorders in children and adolescents to less than 17 percent, from an estimated 20 percent among youth younger than 18 in 1992 (U.S. Department of Health and Human Services, 1991). As of 1997, the summary list of mental health objectives for Healthy People 2000 included reducing suicides to no more than 8.2 per 100,000 youth (aged 15–19) and reducing the incidence of injuries suicide attempts among adolescents to 1.8 percent and, more specifically, to 2.0 percent among female adolescents (U.S. Department of Health and Human Services, 1995). A number of other objectives in the Violent and Abusive Behavior category was to reduce the incidence of physical fighting among adolescents aged 14–17 from a baseline of 137 incidents per 100,000 high school students per month to 110 per 100,000 (U.S. Department of Health and Human Services, 1995).

Though there is extensive research yet to be done in the area of children and adolescent mental health, there is a body of knowledge available to clinicians to assist them in assessing this population when they present with mental health problems. Research based measures guide treatment, which allows the clinician to inform their clients of likely outcomes and even suggest other treatments (Resnick, 1996a, 1996b). Thyer (1995) states for whatever reasons, social workers (and psychologists, psychiatrists, counselors, and so forth) typically did not keep abreast of recent developments in ineffective psychosocial interventions. It is increasingly evident that social workers and other practitioners serving young clients have an ethical and professional obligation to become acquainted with these approaches to practice and provide them as a first-choice treatment whenever appropriate.

The profession itself has an obligation to promote research by its members to further establish empirically based interventions. Research indicates that most mental health professionals including social workers, psychologists, psychiatrist, and counselors never published a single article in any professional or scientific journal over their entire careers. This leads one to question whether they ever engage in the rigorous thinking that professional writing demands (Campbell, 1994). Also it leaves open for discussion whether academia is producing critical thinkers who have been encouraged to develop an empirically based practice (Wodarski & Hilarski, in press).

In the medical world research generally guides practice and many interventions are not available for clinical use until proven effective in the laboratory. This results in protection in the health and welfare of the public (Campbell, 1994). Perhaps mental health professions also should set standards whereby practice guidelines are dictated by empirically proven research before being implemented in practice.

One study done of 1100 mental health workers in community clinics and hospitals indicated that less than 10 percent relied on professional publications in their treatment work (Norris, 1976 as cited in Campbell, 1994). Psychologists in another study were unable to cite any specific research which affected how they practice (Cohen, 1968 as cited in Campbell, 1994). Home and Darveau-Fournier (1982) report a study where only 30 percent of social group workers studied were able to identify any theoretical influences on their work. One additional study examined 416 intake evaluations completed by various mental health professionals. Only one evaluation of relevant research resulted in a treatment rationale that demonstrated an awareness of relevant research (O'Donohue et al., 1988 as cited in Campbell, 1994). This apparent dislike of research by mental health practitioners has direct implications on their practice involving treatment decisions. One study indicates that, in 90 percent of cases that were reviewed, mental health professionals disregarded relevant research and or systematic decision making when choosing assessment procedures, defining treatment goals, and selecting treatment methods (Campbell, 1994). The implications this has for the mental health field is frightening when considering client rights and clinician's ethical respons- ibilities. Campbell (1994) states that practitioners who ignore research are akin to charlatans and faith-healers and may jeopardize the welfare of their patients.

Legal Issues

No doubt social workers and other professionals working without empirically based practices are at risk for increased malpractice suits. Society has begun to demand proof that interventions work (Sanderson, 1995a, 1995b). Campbell (1994) proposes that psychotherapists who fail to stay current with the literature, or to develop appropriate treatment plans, and who encour- age clients' dependency and create imaginary problems invite malpractice litigation.

As social workers, we are held accountable for our professional and personal behaviors. Malpractice suits have increased over the years stemming from a claim of incompetence to sexual misbehavior. Clinicians are not the only ones being held responsible for professional behavior. Universities are being challenged as to their role in educating incompetent practitioners. A lawsuit was filed in Louisiana whereby a client successfully sued her therapist and was awarded 1.7 million dollars. The therapist was a graduate of an educational program with an emphasis in counseling from Louisiana Tech of Education. Now a lawsuit is pending as to whether the college adequately prepared this graduate (Custer, 1994). Is academia adequately preparing students to enter the field as a mental health clinicians? In referring to social work masters programs Hepler and Noble (1990) propose that the quality of social work education ultimately affects practice competence and the social welfare of citizens. Where then does responsibility end for the school and rest with the graduate who is not the practitioner?

The National Association of Social Workers' (NASW, 2006) code of ethics points out the importance of competence in section 1.04. The code reads as follows: "Social Workers should provide services and represent themselves as competent only within the boundaries of their education, training, license, certification, consultation received, supervised experience, or other relevant professional experience." Many practitioners utilize continuing education to enhance their knowledge base.

Continuing education provides providers the practitioner with opportunities to remain current on new research but it also provides more. Houle et al. (1987: 87) state,

> it increases awareness that the appropriate goals broaden out to include all the needs for the growth of a profession, beginning with an awareness of its appropriate mission and continuing through a mastery of both its knowledge base and its methods of treatment, its internal structuring, its code of ethics, its relationships with allied professions, its internal responsibilities to both its clients and its society.

In many states though there are no requirements to maintain a minimal amount of continuing education each year for some professionals. This continuing education must provide the most updated education for providing professionals to function effectively in managed-care environments.

Use of Groups

Cost efficiency and treatment effectiveness are good arguments for group work (Backenstrab et al., 2001; Himle et al., 2001; Morrison, 2001; Randall & Wordarski, 1989). In 1983 three different approaches to family therapy were compared by Christensen, Johnson, Phillips, and Glasgow: a group method, individual mode, and minimal contact with the provision of reading material and brief personal intervention by the worker. Each was provided to improve parent effectiveness with problem children and had multiple measures to evaluate outcomes. Findings indicated that group and individual methods were best and equal to each other with the group condition requiring less than half as much professional time (Randall & Wodarski, 1989).

Toseland and Rivas (2005) report that, the purpose of the group determines each focal area the group will receive. Group work involves the following aspects: in group practice there is a broad range of treatment and task groups; a focus on individual group members, the group as a whole, and the group's environment; application of foundation of knowledge and skills from generalists' social work practice to a broad range of leadership and membership situations. Integration and the use of specialized knowledge and skills are based on a comprehensive assessment of the needs of a particular group; a recognition of the interactional and situational nature of leadership.

Yalom (1995) report a study by Toseland and Siporin that also supports that group therapy is at least as efficacious as individual therapy. This particular study indicated that group therapy was more effective than individual therapy in 25 percent of their studies. In the other 75 percent, there were no significant differences between group and individual therapy. In no study was individual therapy more effective. This indicates that group therapy may be the empirically proven treatment of choice with a certain diagnosis while at the same time being cost-effective for the client, agency, and third party payer.

Evidence-Based Practice

Many evidence based writers emphasize the use of critical-thinking skills for evaluating and using knowledge for practice. All authors agree to the following four principles:

1 Critical thinking is essential to development as a social work professional.
2 Social work practice should be guided by the best available evidence.
3 Social work practitioners have an obligation to monitor client progress.
4 Social work practitioners build their own practice models based on their experience and the experience of others.

Important to their discussion is their attention to the benefits as well as the challenges to using evidence in social work practice.

In their recommendations for the development and incorporation of critical thinking into one's practice, authors have listed eight guiding questions for invoking critical thinking in the examination of various theories of practice:

1 What is the issue or claim being made, in simple and direct language?
2 Are there any ambiguities or a lack of clarity in the claim?
3 What are the underlying value and theory assumptions?
4 Is there indication of any misleading beliefs or faulty reasoning?
5 How good is the evidence presented?
6 Is there any important information missing?
7 Is consideration given to alternative explanations?
8 Are the conclusions reasonable?

In an exemplary chapter on "Science and Evidence-Based Social Work Practice," Thyer and Wodarski mention Persons' (1999) model of practice for the evidence-based practitioner who:

1 Provides informed consent for treatment.
2 Relies on the efficacy data (especially from [randomized controlled trials]).
3 Uses the empirical literature to guide decision-making.
4 Uses a systematic, hypothesis-testing approach to the treatment of each case that:

   (a) Begins with careful assessment,
   (b) Sets clear and measurable treatment goals,

    (c) Develops an individualized formulation and a treatment plan based on the formulation, and

    (d) Monitors progress towards the goals frequently and modifies or ends treatment as needed.

Conclusion

Social workers and other mental health professionals are also receiving pressure from managed care companies to produce empirically based treatment with proven outcomes. Managed care is an inescapable element of mental health services in America today with many private and public insurances now utilizing the cost containment program (Wodarski, 2000) which often places caps on the number of outpatient mental health sessions allowed (Foos et al., 1991). Thyer (1995) states that to the extent that service providers can produce evidence that services provided are well supported by sound clinical research studies, authorizations for such treatment are enhanced. When managed care programs produce incentives for selection of existing demonstrable effective treatments, both the profession and the clients will benefit. As third parties make decisions regarding reimbursement for treatment for clients, practitioners will be forced to demonstrate outcome-based treatments.

As mental health professionals provide service to clients with mental health disorders, it is indeed essential that they provide excellent assessments and match empirically proven treatment to diagnosis. This requires a working knowledge of all sectors of the DSM-IV (American Psychiatric Association, 1994). Also, it demands an ongoing quest for new knowledge and training for the practitioner to enable them to provide the most effective treatment for the clients. Nothing less is ethically acceptable, with less possibility of leading to legal implications. In addition, it is imperative to have an outcome based practice so that clients can access treatment as needed through a third-party gatekeeper called managed care.

The use of research techniques offers the social worker the exciting possibility of evaluating practice on empirical data and not the basis of faith and practice authority. As the demand for competent social workers increases, the training of empirical practitioners will have to be formalized and competency criteria developed. Where practitioners should be trained and what level of skills must be required at each educational degree level are yet to be determined. What are the basic training functions at the undergraduate level, at the master's level, at the doctoral level (Wodarski et al., 1995; Wodarski & Hilarski, in press)? Entrance criteria for students who will become empirical practitioners and appropriate objectives for training must be developed. Also, testing procedures will have to be developed and incorporated into training programs to ensure that practitioners meet appropriate standards. Such an assessment process will ensure that the individuals who call themselves empirical practitioners are really competent to engage in research and development of practice technology (Arkava & Brennen, 1975;

Armitage & Clark, 1975). Furthermore, a new confidence in the change methods being employed should help alleviate the crisis of credibility in social work practice. The incorporation of research can lead only to improvement of services offered to clients through the managed care system.

References

1 Behavioral Medicine and Managed Care: Implications for Social Work Practice

Abeles, N. (1986). Proceedings of the American Psychological Association, for the year 1985: Minutes of the Annual Meeting of the Council of Representatives. *American Psychologist*, 41, 633–663.

Abramson, E. E. (1977). Behavioral approaches to weight control: An updated review. *Behavior Research and Therapy*, 15(4), 355–363.

Agras, W. S. (1982). Behavioral medicine in the 1980s: Non-random connections. *Journal of Consulting and Clinical Psychology*, 50(6), 797–803.

Agras, W. S., Schneider, J. A., Arnow, B., Raeburn, S. D., & Telch C. F. (1989). Cognitive-behavioral treatment with and without exposure plus response prevention in the treatment of bulimia nervosa: A reply to Leitenberg and Rosen. *Journal of Consulting and Clinical Psychology*, 57(6), 778–779.

Baird, K. A., & Rupert, P. A. (2004). Managed care and the independent practice of Psychology. *Professional Psychology: Research and Practice*, 35(2), 185–193.

Bandura, A. (1969). *Principles of behavior modification*. New York: Holt, Rinehart & Winston.

Bandura, A. (1977). *Social learning theory*. Englewood Cliffs, NJ: Prentice-Hall.

Berkman, B. (1996). The emerging health care world: Implications for social work practice and education. *Social Work*, 41(5), 541–551.

Berkman, B., Bedell, D., Parker, E., McCarthy, L., & Rosenbaum C. (1988). Preadmission screening: An efficacy study. *Social Work Health Care*, 13(3), 35–50.

Berwick, D. M., Murphy, J. M., Goldman, P. A., Ware, J. E., Barsky, A. J., & Weinstein, M. C. (1991). Performance of a five-item mental health screening test. *Medical Care*, 29(2), 169–176.

Blanchard, E. B. (1982). Behavioral medicine: Past, present, and future. *Journal of Consulting and Clinical Psychology*, 50(6), 795–796.

Blanchard, E. B., McCoy, G. C., Berger, M., Musso, A., Pallmeyer, T. P., & Gerardi, R., et al. (1989). A controlled comparison of thermal biofeedback and relaxation training in the treatment of essential hypertension IV: Prediction of short-term clinical outcome. *Behavior Therapy*, 20(3), 405–415.

Breslow, L., & Enstrom, J. E. (1980). Persistence of health habits and their relationship to mortality. *Preventive Medicine*, 9, 469–483.

Buxbaum, C. B. (1981). Cost benefit analysis: The mystique versus the reality. *Social Service Review*, 23(3), 226–232.

Callister, R. R., & Wall, J. A., Jr. (2001). Conflict across organizational boundaries: Managed care organizations versus healthcare providers. *Journal of Applied Psychology*, 86(4), 754–763.

Cautela, J. R. (1970a). Covert reinforcement. *Behavior Therapy*, 1(1), 33–50.

Cautela, J. R. (1970b). The treatment of alcoholism by covert sensitization. *Psychotherapy: Theory, Research and Practice*, 7(2), 83–90.

Cautela, J. R. (1970c). Treatment of smoking by covert sensitization. *Psychological Reports*, 26(2), 415–420.

Cautela J. R. (1970d). Covert negative reinforcement. *Journal of Behavior Therapy and Experimental Psychiatry*, 1(4), 273–278.

Cautela, J. R. (1971). Covert extinction. *Behavior Therapy*, 2(2), 192–200.

Cinciripini, P. M., & Floreen, A. (1982). An evaluation of a behavioral program for chronic pain. *Journal of Behavioral Medicine*, 5, 375–388.

Clay, R. A. (2005, February). The changing face of psychology practice. *Monitor on Psychology*, 48–52.

Coulter, M. L., & Hancock, T. (1989). Integrating social work and public health education: A clinical model. *Health Social Work*, 14(3), 157–164.

Cummings, J. W. (1992). Psychologists in the medical-surgical setting: Some reflections. *Professional Psychology: Research and Practice*, 23(2), 76–79.

Cummings, N. (1995). Impact of managed care on employment and training: A primer for survival. *Professional Psychology: Research and Practice*, 26, 10–15.

Cummings, N. A., Pallak, M. S., & Cummings, J. L. (Eds.) (1996). *Surviving the demise of solo practice: Mental health practitioners prospering in the era of managed care*. Madison, CT: Psychosocial Press.

Daniels, J. A., Alva, L. A., & Olivares, S. (2002). Graduate training for managed care: A national survey of psychology and social work programs. *Professional Psychology: Research and Practice*, 33(6), 587–590.

Dingfelder, S. F. (2006, June). Taking it 20 minutes at a time. *Monitor on Psychology*, 20–21.

Dulmus C., & Wodarski, J. S. (1996). Assessment and effective treatments of childhood psychopathology: Responsibilities and implications for practice. *Journal of Child and Adolescent Group Therapy*, 6(2), 75–99.

el-Askari, G., Freestone, J., Irizarry, C., Kraut, K. L., Mashiyama, S. T. Morgan, M. A., et al. (1998). The healthy neighborhoods project: A local health department's role in catalyzing community development. *Health Education Behavior*, 25(2), 146–159.

Eysenck, H. J. (1988). Health's character. *Psychology Today*, 22(12), 28–35.

Findlay, S. (1998). 85% of American workers using HMO's. *USA Today*, January 20 p. 3a.

Fischer, J. (1971). A framework for the analysis and comparison of clinical theories of induced change. *Social Service Review*, 45(4), 440–454.

Fischer, J. (1978). *Effective casework practice*. New York: McGraw-Hill.

Flowers, J. V, Booraem, C. D., & Schwartz, B. (1993). Impact of computerized rapid assessment instruments on counselors and client outcome. *Computers in Human Services*, 10(2), 9–18.

Friedman, R., Sobel, D., Myers, P., Caudill, M., & Benson, H. (1995). Behavioral medicine, clinical health psychology and cost offset. *Health Psychology*, 14, 509–518.

Gray, G., Brody, D., & Johnson, D. (2005). The evolution of behavioral primary care. *Professional Psychology: Research and Practice*, 36(2), 123–129.

Gross, A. M. (1980). Appropriate cost reporting: An indispensable link to accountability. *Administration in Social Work*, 1(3), 31–41.

Gross, A. M., Gross, J., & Einsenstein-Naveh, A. R. (1983). Defining the role of the social worker in primary health care. *Health & Social Work*, 8, 174–181.

Hilarski, C., & Wodarski, J. S. (2001). The effective social worker. *Journal of Human Behavior in the Social Environment*, 4(1), 19–38.

Hookey, P. (1979). Cost-benefit evaluations in primary health care. *Health & Social Work*, 4, 151–167.

Hudson, W. W. (1982). *The clinical measurement package: A field manual*. Homewood, IL: Dorsey Press.

Jeffery, R. W. (1989). Risk behaviors and health: Contrasting individual and population perspectives. *American Psychologist*, 44(9), 1194–1202.

Kent, A. J., & Hersen, M. (2000). An overview of managed mental health care: Past, present, and future. In A. J. Kent & M. Hersen (Eds.), *A psychologist's proactive guide to managed mental health care* (pp. 3–19). Mahwah, NJ: Erlbaum.

Kersting, K. (2005a, September). A showcase for the mind-body connection. *Monitor on Psychology*, 36(8), 42.

Kersting, K. (2005b, February). Health-care calling: Psychologists' roles in health care are well established and growing. *Monitor on Psychology*, 56–58.

Krantz D. S., & Blumenthal, J. A. (Eds.) (1987). *Behavioral assessment and management of cardiovascular disorders*. Sarasota, FL: Professional Resource Exchange.

Kroenke, K., & Mangelsdorf, A. (1989). Common symptoms in primary care: Incidence, evaluation, therapy and outcome. *American Journal of Medicine*, 86, 262–266.

Lally, R. J., Mangione, P. L., & Honig, A. S. (1988). *The Syracuse University Family Development Research Program: Long-range impact on an early intervention with low-income children and their families*. Norwood, NJ: Ablex Publishers.

Law, B. (2006, May). Design for whole-person care: Integrating psychology into primary medical care requires psychologists to act nationally and locally. *Monitor on Psychology*, 42–43.

Leukefeld, C. G. (1989). Psychosocial issues in dealing with AIDS. *Hospital Community Psychiatry*, 40(5), 454–455.

Levin, H. M. (1983). *Cost effectiveness: A primer. In new perspectives in evaluation* (Vol. 4). Beverly Hills, CA: Sage Publications.

Levy, R. L. (1987). Compliance and clinical practice. In J. Blumenthal and D. McKee (Eds.), *Applications in behavioral medicine and health psychology: A clinician's source book* (pp. 567–587). Sarasota, FL: Professional Resource Exchange.

Liskow, B., Campbell, J., Nickel, E., & Powell, B. (1995). Validity of the CAGE questionnaire in screening for alcohol dependence in a walk-in (triage) clinic. *Journal of Studies on Alcohol*, 156(3), 227–281.

McClelland, D. C. (1989). Motivational factors in health and disease. *American Psychologist*, 44(4), 675–683.

MacLeod, J. (1995). *Ain't no makin' it: Aspirations and attainment in a low-income neighborhood*. Boulder, CO: Westview Press.

McMahon, M. O. (1984). *The general method of social work practice*. Englewood Cliffs, NJ: Prentice-Hall.

Marshack, E., Davidson, K., & Mizahi, T. (1988). Preparation of social workers for a changing health care environment. *Health Social Work*, 13(3), 226–233.

Masia, C. L., Anderson, C. M., McNeil, D. W., & Hawkins, R. P. (1997). Managed care and graduate training: A call for action. *Behavior Therapist*, 20, 145–148.

Matthews, K. (2005). Psychological perspectives on the development of coronary heart disease. *American Psychologist*, 783–796.

Meyers, L. (2006, June). Still a system in need of repairs. *Monitor on Psychology*, 50–51.

Mizrahi, T. (1993). Managed care and managed competition: A primer for social work. *Health & Social Work*, 18(2), 86–91.

Muehrer, P. (1996). Economic analysis in applied psychosocial research. *NIMH Psychotherapy and Rehabilitation Research Bulletin*, 5, 10.

Munsey, C. (2006, May). Psychology can help solve America's health-care crisis: The public needs psychology's insights on changing behavior to lead healthier lives. *Monitor on Psychology*, 36–38.

Narrow, W., Reiger, D., Rae. D., Manderscheid, R., & Locke, B. (1993). Use of services by persons with mental and addictive disorders: Findings from the National Institute of Mental Health Epidemiologic Catchments Area Program. *Archives of General Psychiatry*, 50, 95–107.

Pace, T., Chaney, J., Mullins, L., & Olson, R. (1995). Psychological consultation with primary care physicians: Obstacles and opportunities in the medical setting. *Professional Psychology: Research and Practice*, 26(2), 123–131.

Packard, E. (2005, December). From basic research to health-care messages: Improved public health is a priority for many APA Div. 8 social psychologists. *Monitor on Psychology*, 84–85.

Pelosi, N. (1996). Reducing risks of mental disorders. *American Psychologist*, 51(11), 1128–1129.

Pinkerton, S., Hughes, N., & Wenrich, W. (1982). *Behavioral medicine: Clinical applications*. New York: Wiley.

Pomerleau, O. F. (1982). A discourse on behavioral medicine: Current status and future trends. *Journal of Consulting and Clinical Psychology*, 50(6), 1030–1039.

Provence, S., & Naylor, A. (1983). *Working with disadvantaged parents and their children: Scientific and practical issues*. New Haven, CT: Yale University Press.

Rains, J. W., & Erickson, G. P. (1997). Putting prevention into practice. *Journal of Professional Nursing*, 13(2), 124–128.

Rapp-Paglicci, L., Dulmus, C., Wodarski, J., & Feit, M. (2000). Screening of substance abuse in public welfare protective service clients: A comparative study of rapid assessment instruments vs. the SASSI. Invited abstract published in *Epikrisis*, 11(3), 2.

Raw, S. D. (1999). Does mental health managed care violate federal antitrust laws? [An interview with Joseph R. Sahid, Esq.] *Behavior Therapist*, 22(3), 53–67.

Resnick, C., & Tighe, E. G. (1997). The role of multidisciplinary community clinics in managed care systems. *Social Work*, 42(1), 91–99.

Rieger, D., Narrow, W., Rae. D., Manderscheid, R, Locke, B., & Goodwin, F. (1993). The de facto US mental and addictive disorders service system: Epidemiologic Catchments Area prospective 1 year prevalence rates of disorders and services. *Archives of General Psychiatry*, 50, 85–94.

Rittner, B., & Wodarski, J. S. (1995). Clinical instruments: Assessing and treating children and families. *Early Child Development and Care*, 106, 43–58.

Robinson, P. (1995). New territory for the behavior therapist: Hello depressed patients in primary care! *The Behavior Therapist*, 18, 149–153.

Robinson, N. S., Garber, J., & Hilsman, R. (1995). Cognitions and stress: Direct and moderating effects on depressive versus externalizing symptoms during the junior high school transition. *Journal of Abnormal Psychology*, 104, 453–463.

Sanchez, L. M., & Turner, S. M. (2003). Practicing psychology in the era of managed care: Implications for practice and training. *American Psychology*, 58(2), 116–129.

Schaible, T., Thomlinson, R., & Susan, P. (2004). The discipline of managing value in collaborative healthcare. *Families, Systems, & Health*, 22(3), 376–382.

Shannon, M. T. (1989). Health promotion and illness prevention: A biopsychosocial perspective. *Health and Social Work*, 14(1), 32–40.

Sledge, W. H., Tebes, J., Rakfeldt, J., Davidson, L., Lyons, L., & Druss, B. (1996). Day hospital/crisis respite care vs. inpatient care, Part E: Service utilization and costs. *American Journal of Psychiatry*, 153, 1074–1083.

Smith, G., Rost, K., & Kashner, T. (1995). A trial of the effect of a standardized psychiatric consultation on health outcomes and costs in somaticizing patients. *Archives of General Psychiatry*, 52, 238–243.

Stoesz, D. (1986). Corporate health care and social welfare. *Health and Social Work*, 11(3), 165–172.

Stokey, E., & Zeckhauser, R. (1978). *A primer for policy analysis* (pp. 135–137). New York: W. Norton & Co.

Streever, K. L., Wodarski, J. S., & Lindsey, E. W. (1984). Assessing client change in human service agencies. *Family Therapy*, 11(2), 163–173.

Strosahl, K. (1994). Entering the new frontier of managed mental health care: Gold mines and land mines. *Cognitive and Behavioral Practice*, I, 5–23.

Strosahl, K. (1995). Behavior therapy 2000: A perilous journey. *The Behavior Therapist*, 75, 130–133.

Stuart, R. B. (1967). Behavioral control of overeating. *Behavior Research and Therapy*, 5(4), 357–365.

Sultz, H. A., & Young, K. M. (1997). *Health care USA: Understanding its organization and delivery*. New York: Aspen Publishers.

Taylor, S. E. (1999). Health psychology: Challenges for the future. In *Health Psychology* (pp. 470–489). New York: McGraw-Hill.

Thyer, B. A., & Wodarski, J. S. (Eds.) (1998). *Handbook of empirical social work practice, Volume1: Mental disorders*. Hoboken, NJ: John Wiley & Sons.

Ugland, J. H. (1989). Health as a value: Implications of practice. *Professional Psychology: Research and Practice*, 20(6), 415–416.

Wilson, G. T., Franks, C. M., Kendall, P. C., & Foreyt, J. P. (1987). Behavioral medicine [Review of Behavior Therapy]. *Theory and Practice*, 11, 155–186.

Wodarski, J. S. (1980). Procedures for the maintenance and generalization of achieved behavioral change. *Journal of Sociology and Social Welfare*, 7(2), 298–311.

Wodarski, J. S. (1985). *Introduction to human behavior*. Austin, TX: PRO-ED.

Wodarski, J. S. (1995). Guidelines for building research centers in schools of social work. *Research on Social Work Practice*, 5(3), 383–398.

Wodarski, J. S. (1997). *Empirical practice: An introduction*. New York: Springer.

Wodarski, J. S. (2000). The role for social workers in the managed health care system: A model for empirically based psychosocial interventions. *Crisis Intervention and Time Limited Treatment*, 6(2), 109–139.

Wodarski, J. S., & Bagarozzi, D. A. (1979). *Behavioral social work*. New York: Human Services Press.

Wodarski, J. S., & Dziegielewski, S. (2002). *Human behavior in the social environment: An empirical approach*. New York: Springer.

Wodarski, J. S., & Feldman. R. A. (1973). The research practicum: A beginning formulation of process and educational objectives. *International Social Work*, 16(4), 42–48.

Wodarski, J. S., Rapp-Paglicci, L. A., Dulmus, C. N., & Jongsma, A. E., Jr. (2001). *The social work and human services treatment planner*. New York: John Wiley & Sons.

Wodarski, L. A., & Wodarski, J. S. (2004). Prevention and treatment of childhood and adolescent obesity. In L. A. Rapp-Paglicci, C. Dulmus, & J. S. Wodarski (Eds.), *Handbook of preventive interventions for children and adolescents* (pp. 301–320). Hoboken, NJ: John Wiley.

Wodarski, J. S., Wodarski, L. A., Nixon, S. C., & Mackie, C. (1991). Behavioral medicine: An emerging field of social work practice. *Journal of Health & Social Policy*, 3(1), 19–43.

2   The Integrated Service Delivery System

Dulmus, C. N., & Wodarski, J. (1997). Prevention of childhood mental disorders: A literature review reflecting hope and a vision for the future. *Child & Adolescent Social Work Journal*, 14(3), 181 198.

Flowers, J., Booraem, C., & Schwartz, B. (1993). Impact of computerized rapid assessment instruments on counselors and client outcomes. *Computers in Human Services*, 25(2), 304–305.

Hays, R., Hill, L., Gillogly, J., & Lewis, M. (1993) Response times for the CAGE, Short-MAST, and Jellinek Alcohol Scales. *Behavior Research Methods, Instruments & Computer*, 25(2), 304–307.

Keigher, S. M. (1997). What role for social work in the new health care practice paradigm? *Health & Social Work*, 22(22), 149–155.

Kroenke, K., & Mangelsdorf, A. (1989). Common symptoms in primary care: Incidence, evaluation, therapy, and outcome. *American Journal of Medicine*, 86, 262–266.

McMahon, R. (1984). Behavioral checklists and rating scales. In T. H. Ollendick & M. Hersen (Eds.), *Child behavior assessment: Principles and procedures* (pp. 80–105). New York: Pergamon.

Rieger, D., Narrow, W., Rae, D., Manderscheid, R., Locke, B., & Goodwin, F. (1993). The de facto US mental and addictive disorders service delivery system: Epidemiological Catchment Area prospective 1-year prevalence rates of disorders and services. *Archives of General Psychiatry*, 50, 238–243.

Rittner, B., & Wodarski, J. S. (1995). Clinical instruments: Assessing and treating children and families. *Early Child Development and Care*, 106, 43–58.

Smith, G., Rost, K., & Kashner, T. (1995). A trial of the effect of a standardized psychiatric consultation on health outcomes and costs in somaticizing patients. *Archives of General Psychiatry*, 52, 238–243.

Streever, K., Wodarski, J., & Lindsey, E. (1984). Assessing client change in human service agencies. *Family Therapy*, 11, 163–173.

3   Managed Care, Assessment Instruments, and Helping Professionals

Bachman, S. S., Drainoni, M. L., & Tobias, C. (2004). Medicaid managed care, substance abuse treatment, and people with disabilities: Review of the literature. *Health and Social Work*, 29(3), 189–196.

Beresford, T. P., Blow, P. C., Hill, E., Singer, K., & Lucey, M. R. (1990). Comparison of AGE questionnaire and computer-assisted laboratory profiles in screening for covert alcoholism. *Lancet*, 1, 325–328.

Berkman, B. (1996). The emerging health care world: Implications for social work practice and education. *Social Work*, 41(5), 541–551.

Berwick, D. M., Murphy, J. M., Goldman, P. A., Ware, J. E., Barsky, A. L., & Weinstein, M. C. (1991). Performance of a five-item mental health screening test. *Medical Care*, 29(2), 169–176.

DeAngelis, T. (2005). Shaping evidence-based practice. *Monitor on Psychology*, 36(3), 26–31.

Elmore, D. (2006, June). An aging America: Psychologists are assisting policy-makers in meeting the needs of older Americans. *Monitor on Psychology*, 82–83.

Ewing, J. A. (1984). Detecting alcoholism, the CAGE questionnaire. *Journal of the American Medical Association*, 252, 1905–1907.

Ewing, J. A., & Rouse, B. A. (1970). Identifying the hidden alcoholic. Paper presented at the 29th International Congress on Alcohol and Drug Dependence. Sydney, Australia.

Gibelman, M., & Mason, S. (2002). Treatment choices in a managed care environment: A multi-disciplinary exploration. *Clinical Social Work Journal*, 30(2), 199–214.

Greene, R. R., & Sullivan, W. P. (2004). Putting social work values into action: Use of the ecological perspective with older adults in the managed care arena. *Journal of Gerontological Social Work*, 42(3/4), 131–150.

Gross, A. M., Gross, L., & Eisenstein-Naveh, A. R. (1983). Defining the role of the social worker in primary health care. *Health & Social Work*, 8, 174–181.

Gureje, O., & Obikoya, B. (1990). The GHQ-12 as a screening tool in a primary care setting. *Social Psychiatry and Psychiatric Epidemiology*, 25(5), 276–280.

Hays, R. D., Merz, L. P., & Nicholas, R. (1995). Response burden, reliability, and validity of the CAGE, short MAST and AUDIT alcohol screening measures. *Behavior Research Methods, Instruments, & Computers*, 27(2), 277–280.

Hookey, P. (1979). Cost-benefit evaluations in primary health care. *Health & Social Work*, 4, 151–167.

Hudson, W. W. (1990). *The multi-problem screening inventory*. Tempe, AZ: WALMYR Publishing Co.

Hudson, W. W., & McMurtry, S. L. (1997). Comprehensive assessment in social work practice: The multi-problem screening inventory. *Research on Social Work Practice*, 7(1), 79–98.

Kane, M. N., Hamlin, E. R., & Hawkins, W. E. (2003). Investigating correlates of clinical social worker's attitudes toward managed care. *Social Work in Health Care*, 36(4), 101–119.

Kapur, R. L., Kapur, M., & Carstairs, G. M. (1984). Indian psychiatric survey schedule. *Social Psychiatry*, 9, 71–76.

Kiesler, C. A. (2000). The next wave of change for psychology and mental health services in the health care revolution. *American Psychologist*, 55(5), 481–487.

Lairson, D. R., Harlow, K., Cobb, J., Harrist, R., Martin, D. W., Ramby, R., et al. (1992). Screening for patients with alcohol problems: Severity of patients identified by the CAGE. *Journal of Drug Education*, 22(4), 337–352.

Law, B. M. (2006, June). Early intervention benefits heavier low birth-weight babies longer. *Monitor on Psychology*, 15, 15.

Liskow, B., & Campbell, J. (1995). Validity of the CAGE questionnaire in screening for alcohol dependence in a walk-in (triage) clinic. *Journal of Studies on Alcohol*, 56(3), 277–281.

Mari, J. J., & Williams, P. (1985). A comparison of the validity of two psychiatric screening questionnaires (GHQ-12 and SRQ-20) in Brazil, using relative operating characteristic (ROC) analysis. *Psychological Medicine*, 15, 651–659.

Mayfield, D., McLeod, G., & Hall, P. (1974). The CAGE questionnaire: Validation of a new alcoholism screening instrument. *American Journal of Psychiatry*, 131, 1121–1123.

Mizrahi, T. (1993). Unmanaged care and managed competition: A primer for social work. *Health & Social Work*, 18, 86–91.

Munson, C. E. (1996). Autonomy and managed care in clinical social work practice. *Smith College Studies in Social Work*, 66(3), 241–260.

Resnick, C., & Tighe, E. G. (1997). The role of multidisciplinary community clinics in managed care systems. *Social Work*, 42(1), 91–98.

Ross, H., & Tisdall, G. (1994). Identification of alcohol disorders at a university mental health center, using the CAGE. *Journal of Alcohol and Drug Education*, 39(3), 119–126.

Shera, W. (1996). Managed care and people with severe mental illness: Challenges and opportunities for social work. *Health and Social Work*, 21(3), 196–202.

Shortell, S. M., Gillies, R. R., & Devers, K. J. (1995). Reinventing the American hospital. *Milbank Quarterly*, 73, 131–160.

Van Hemert, A. M., Heijer, M. D., Vorstenbosch, M., & Bolk, J. H. (1995). Detecting psychiatric disorders in medical practice using the General Health Questionnaire. Why do cut off scores vary? *Psychological Medicine*, 25(1), 165–170.

Watson, C. G., Debra, E., Fox, K. L., & Ewing, J. W. (1995). Comparative concurrent validities of five alcoholism measures in a psychiatric hospital. *Journal of Clinical Psychology*, 51, 676–684.

Wodarski, J. S. (1997). *Research methods for clinical social workers: Empirical practice*. New York: Springer Publishing Company.

4 Development of Managed Information Systems for Human Services: A Practical Guide

Boyd L. H., Jr., Hylton, J. H., & Price, S. V. (1978). Computers in social work practice: A review. *Social Work*, 23, 368–371.

Butler, D. L. (1986). Statistics packages. *Contemporary Psychology*, 31, 485–487.

Carlson, R. W. (1985). Connecting clinical information processing with computer support. *Computers in Human Services*, 1, 51–66.

Cash, K. (1983). Simulation and gaming in social work education: A projection. *Journal of Education for Social Work*, 19, 111–118.

Catherwood, H. R. (1974). A management information system for social services. *Public Welfare*, 32, 56–61.

Chamberlin, J. (2005, November). Prize-winning paper explores the ethics of marketing to children. *Monitor on Psychology*, 16.

Dziegielewski, S. F. (2004). *The changing face of health care social work*. New York: Springer Publishing Company.

Faherty, V. E. (1983). Simulation and gaming in social work education: A projection. *Journal of Education for Social Work*, 19, 111–118.

Faul, A. C., & Hudson, W. W. (1997, November). The index of drug involvement: A partial validation. *Social Work*, 42(6), 565–572.

Friedman, T. L. (2006). *The world is flat: A brief history of the twenty-first century* (updated and expanded edition). New York: Farrar, Straus & Giroux.

Fuller, T. K. (1970). Computer utility in social work. *Social Casework*, 51, 606–611.

Geiss, G. R., & Viswanathan, N. (1986). *The human edge information technology and helping people.* New York: The Haworth Press.

Goplerud, E. N., Walfish, S., & Broskowski, A. (1985). Weathering the cuts: A Delphi survey on surviving cutbacks in community mental health. *Community Mental Health Journal*, 21, 14–27.

Green, M. S. (1984). Computer resources and terminology: A brief introduction. *Counselor Education and Supervision*, 24, 133–141.

Hartmann, D. P., Wood, D. D., & Shigetomi, C. C. (1981). Guidelines for maintaining a productive clinical research career. *Behavioral Assessment*, 3, 273–282.

Hedlund, J. L., Vieweg, B. W., & Cho, D. W. (1985). Mental health computing in the 1980s: I. General information systems and clinical documentation. *Computers in Human Services*, 1, 3–33.

Hosford, R. E., & Johnson, M. E. (1983). A comparison of self observation, self-modeling, and practice without video feedback for improving counselor-interviewing behaviors. *Counselor Education and Supervision*, 23, 62–70.

Hosie, T. W., & Smith, C. W. (1984). Piloting. *Counselor Education and Supervision*, 24, 176–185.

Howing, P. T., Wodarski, J. S., Gaudin, J. M., Jr., & Kurtz, P. D. (1989). Clinical assessment instruments in the treatment of child abuse and neglect. *Early Child Development and Care*, 42, 71–84.

Hudson, W. W. (1992). *The WALMYR assessment scales scoring manual.* Tempe, AZ: WALMYR Publishing Company.

Iuppa, N. V. (1984). *A practical guide to interactive video design.* White Plains, NY: Knowledge Industry Publications.

Kreuger, L. W., & Ruckdeschel, R. (1985). Microcomputers in social service settings: Research applications. *Social Work*, 30, 219–224.

Lewis, J., & Gibson, F. (1977). The teaching of some social work skills: Towards a skill laboratory. *British Journal of Social Work*, 7, 189–209.

Lichtenburg, J. W., Hummel, T. J., & Shaffer, W. F. (1984). CLIENT 1: A computer simulation for use in counselor education and research. *Counselor Education and Research*, 24, 176–185.

Meldman, M. J., Harris, D., Pellicore, R. J., & Johnson, E. L. (1977). A computer-assisted, goal oriented psychiatric progress note system. *American Journal of Psychiatry*, 134, 38–41.

Meinert, R. G. (1972). Simulation technology: A potential tool for social work education. *Journal of Education for Social Work*, 8, 50–59.

Mullen, E. J., & Dumpson, I. R. (1972). *Evaluation of social intervention.* San Francisco, CA: Jossey-Bass.

Mutschler, E., & Jayaratne, S. (1994). Integration of information technology and single-system designs: Issues and promises. *Journal of Social Service Research*, 18(1/2), 121–145.

Newmark, C. S. (1985). *Major psychological assessment instruments, Volume 2.* Needham Heights, MA: Allyn & Bacon.

Nugent, W. R., Sieppert, J. D., & Hudson, W. W. (2001). *Practice evaluation for the 21st century.* Belmont, CA: Brooks/Cole-Thomson Learning.

Parker-Oliver, D., & Demiris, G. (2006). Social work informatics. A new speciality. *Social Work*, 51(2), 127–134.

Phillips, S. D. (1984a). Contributions and limitations in the use of computers in counselor training. *Counselor Education and Supervision*, 24, 130–132.

Phillips, S. D. (1984b). Computers as counseling and training tools. *Counselor Education and Supervision*, 24, 186–192.

Pribble, R. (1985). Enter the videodisc. *Training*, 3, 62–70.

Rapp, C. A. (1984). Information, performance, and the human service manager of the 1980s: Beyond "housekeeping." *Administration in Social Work*, 8, 69–80.

Rinn, R. C., & Vernon, J. C. (1975). Process evaluation of outpatient treatment in a community mental health center. *Journal of Behavior Therapy and Experimental Psychiatry*, 6, 5–11.

Rittner, B., & Wordarski, J. S. (1995). Clinical assessment instruments in the treatment of child abuse and neglect. *Early Child Development and Care*, 106, 43–58.

Ruggiero, K. J., Resnick, H. S., Acierno, R., Carpenter, M. J., Kilpatrick, D. G., Coffey, S. F., et al. (2006, June). Internet-based intervention for mental health and substance use problems in disaster-affected populations: A pilot feasibility study. *Behavior Therapy*, 37(2), 190–205.

Shay, C. (1980). Simulations in the classroom: An appraisal. *Educational Technology*, 20, 11–15.

Tornatzky, L. G., Eveland, J. D., Boylan, M. G., Hetzner, E. C., Johnson, D., Roitman, D., et al. (1983). *The process of technological innovation: Reviewing the literature*. Washington, DC: National Science Foundation.

Wagman, M., & Kerber, K. W. (1984). Computer-assisted counseling: Problems and prospects. *Counselor Education and Supervision*, 24, 142–154.

White, A. (1984, October). A sample of counselor educators about microcomputers. Paper presented at the annual meeting of the Northern Rocky Mountain Educational Research Association.

Wodarski, J. S. (1981). *Role of research in clinical practice*. Baltimore, MD: University Park Press.

Wodarski, J. S. (1986). The application of computer technology to enhance the effectiveness of family therapy. *Family Therapy*, 13, 5–13.

Wodarski, J. S., & Bagarozzi, D. (1979). *Behavioral social work*. New York: Human Sciences Press.

Wodarski, J. S., Bricout, J., & Smokowski, P. R. (1996). Making interactive videodisc computer simulation accessible and practice relevant. *Journal of Teaching in Social Work*, 13(1/2), 15–26.

5 Psychosocial Treatment Configurations

Allen, S. F., & Tracy, E. M. (2004). Revitalizing the role of home visiting by school social workers. *Children and Schools*, 26(4), 197–208.

American Psychological Association (1995). *Template for developing guidelines: Interventions for mental disorders and psychosocial aspects of physical disorders*. Washington, DC: American Psychological Association.

Ammerman, R. T., Last, C. G., & Hersen, M. (1993). *Handbook of prescriptive treatments for children and adolescents*. Needham Heights, MA: Allyn & Bacon.

Anderson-Butcher, D., Newsome, W. S., & Nay, S. (2003, July). Social skills intervention during elementary school recess: A visual analysis. *Children & Schools*, 25(3), 135–146.

Arnold, L. E. (1995). Some nontraditional psychosocial treatments for children and adolescents: Critique and proposed screening principles—unconventional and or innovative [Special Issue]. *Psychosocial Treatment Research.*

Baez, A. (2003). A group approach to fostering self-cohesion and developmental progression in female adolescent group home residents. *Child and Adolescent Social Work Journal*, 20(5), 351–373.

Behrens, M. L., & Ackerman, N. W. (1956). The home visit as an aid in family diagnosis and therapy. *Social Casework*, 37(1), 11–19.

Benight, C. C., & Bandura, A. (2004). Social cognitive theory of posttraumatic recovery: The role of perceived self-efficacy. *Behaviour Research and Therapy*, 42(10), 1129–1148.

Beutler, L. E., & Kendall, P. C. (1995). Introduction to the special section: The case for training in the provision of psychological therapy. *Journal of Consulting and Clinical Psychology*, 63(2), 179–181.

Bloom, J. R., Stewart, S. L., Johnston, M., Banks, P., & Fobair, P. (2001). Sources of support and the physical and mental well-being of young women with breast cancer. *Social Science and Medicine*, 53, 1513–1524.

Bond, G. R., McGrew, J. H., & Fekete, D. M. (1995). Assertive outreach for frequent users of psychiatric hospitals: A meta-analysis. *Journal of Mental Health Administration*, 22(1), 4–16.

Chambless, D. L. (1996). In defense of dissemination of empirically supported psychological interventions. *Clinical Psychology: Science and Practice*, 3(3), 230–235.

Chappel, J. N., & Daniels, R. S. (1970). Home visiting in a black urban ghetto. *American Journal of Psychiatry*, 126(10), 1455–1460.

Csiernick, R. C., & Troller, J. (2002). Evaluating the effectiveness of a relapse prevention group. *Journal of Social Work Practice in the Addictions*, 2(2), 29–37.

Davidson, G. S., & Neale, J. M. (1974). The effects of signal-noise similarity on visual information processing of schizophrenics. *Journal of Abnormal Psychology*, 83(6), 683–686.

Devine, E. C., & Westlake, S. K. (1995). The effects of psychoeducational care provided to adults with cancer: Meta-analysis of 116 studies. *Oncology Nursing Forum*, 22, 1369–1381.

Dulmus, C. N., & Wodarski, J. S. (1996). Assessment and effective treatments of childhood psychopathology: Responsibilities and implications for practice. *The Journal of Child and Adolescent Group Therapy*, 6(2), 75–99.

Durlak, J. A. (1979). Comparative effectiveness of paraprofessional and professional helpers. *Psychological Bulletin*, 86, 80–92.

Emrick, C. D., Lassen, C. L., & Edwards, M. T. (1977). Nonprofessional peers as therapeutic agents. In A. S. Gurman & A. M. Razin (Eds.), *Effective psychotherapy* (pp. 12–161). New York: Pergamon Press.

Fennell, M. J. (2004). Depression, low self-esteem and mindfulness. *Behaviour Research and Therapy*, 42(9), 1053–1057.

Faver, C. A. (2004). Relational spirituality and social caregiving. *Social Work*, 49(2), 241–249.

Fawzy, F. I., & Fawzy, N. W. (1998). Group therapy in the cancer setting. *Journal of Psychosomatic Research*, 45, 191–200.

Fisher, J. (1978). Does anything work? *Journal of Social Service Research*, 1(3), 215–243.

Freeman, R. D. (1967). The home visit in child psychiatry: Its usefulness in diagnosis and training. *Journal of American Academy of Child Psychiatry*, 6, 276–279.

Fuhriman A., & Burlingame, G. M. (1994). Measuring small group process: A methodological application of chaos theory. *Small Group Research*, 25(4), 502–519.

Garfield, S. L. (1971). Research on client variables in psychotherapy. In A. Berg & S. Garfield (Eds.), *Handbook of psychotherapy and behavior change* (pp. 271–298). New York: John Wiley & Sons.

Garfield, S. L., & Bergin, A. E. (1986). Introduction and historical overview. In S. L. Garfield & A. E. Bergin (Eds.), *Handbook of psychotherapy and behavior change* (3rd ed.). New York: John Wiley & Sons.

Giles, T. R. (1993). *Handbook of effective psychotherapy*. New York: Plenum Press.

Giles, T. R., Prial, E. M., & Neims, D. M. (1993). Evaluating psychotherapies: A comparison of effectiveness. *International Journal of Mental Health*, 22(2), 43–65.

Glass, C. R., & Arnkoff, D. B. (1992). Behavior therapy. In D. K. Freedheim, H. Freudenberger, D. R. Peterson, J. W. Kessler, H. H. Strupp, S. B. Messer, et al. (Eds.), *History of psychotherapy: A century of change* (pp. 587–628). Washington, DC: American Psychological Association.

Glenn, M., & Kunnes, R. (1973). *Repression or revolution? Therapy in the United States today*. Oxford, UK: Harper Colophon.

Goldfried, M. R., Greenberg, L. S., & Marmar, C. (1990). Individual psychotherapy: Process and outcome. *Annual Review of Psychology*, 41, 659–688.

Gorey, K. M. (1996). Effectiveness of social work intervention research: Internal versus external evaluations. *Social Work Research*, 20(2), 119–128.

Gorey, K. M., Thyer, B. A., & Pawluck, D. E. (1998). Differential effectiveness of prevalent social work practice models: A meta-analysis. *Social Work*, 43(3), 269–278.

Gurman, A. S., & Razin, A. M. (Eds.) (1977). *Effective psychotherapy*. New York: Plenum Press.

Halla, P. L., & Tarrier, N. (2002). *The cognitive-behavioural treatment of low-self esteem in psychotic patients: A pilot study*. Manchester, UK: Trafford Healthcare NHS Trust.

Harrison, D. F., Wodarski, J. S., & Thyer, B. A. (1992). *Cultural diversity and social work practice*. Springfield, IL: Charles Thompson Publishers.

Harrison, D. F., Wodarski, J. S., & Thyer, B. A. (in press). *Cultural diversity and social work practice* (3rd ed.). Springfield, IL: Charles Thompson Publishers.

Henggeler, S. W., Schoenwald, S. K., & Pickrel, S. G. (1995). Multisystemic therapy: Bridging the gap between university- and community-based treatment. *Journal of Consulting and Clinical Psychology*, 63(5), 709–717.

Hilarski, C., & Wodarski, J. S. (2001). The effective social worker. *Journal of Human Behavior in the Social Environment*, 4(1), 19–39.

Hogart, G. E., Goldberg, S. C., Schooler, N. R., & Ulrich, R. F. (1974). Drug and sociotherapy in the aftercare of schizophrenic patients. II. Two-year relapse rates. *Archives of General Psychiatry*, 31(5), 603–608.

Hollis, F. (1972). *Casework: A psychosocial therapy* (2nd ed.). New York: Random House.

Institute of Medicine (1989). *Assessment of diagnostic technology in health care. Rationale, methods, problems, and directions*. Washington, DC: National Academy Press. Reprinted with permission from the National Academy of Sciences, courtesy of the National Academies Press, Washington, DC.

Johnstone, B., Frank, R. G., Belar, C., Berk, S., Bieliauskas, L. A., Bigler, E. D. et al. (1995). Psychology in health care: Future directions. *Professional Psychology: Research and Practice*, 26, 341–365.

Jones, L. V. (2001, May). Enhancing psychosocial competence among black women through an innovative psycho-educational group intervention. *Dissertation Abstracts International, A: The Humanities and Social Sciences*, 61(11), 4550-A, Social Services Abstracts.

Kazdin, A. E. (1975a). Covert modeling, imagery assessment, and assertive behavior. *Journal of Consulting and Clinical Psychology*, 43(5), 716–724.

Kazdin, A. E. (1975b). Characteristics and trends in applied behavior analysis. *Journal of Applied Behavior Analysis*, 8(3), 332.

Laws, D. R. (1999, March). Relapse prevention: The state of the art. *Journal of Interpersonal Violence*, 14(3), 285–302.

Levine, M., & Perkins, D. V. (1987). *Principles of community psychology: Perspective and applications*. New York: Oxford University Press.

MacDonald, G., Sheldon, B., & Gillespie, J. (1992). Contemporary studies of the effectiveness of social work. *British Journal of Social Work*, 22(6), 615–643.

Matto, H. C. (2001, January). Investigating the clinical utility of the draw-a-person: Screening procedure for emotional disturbance (DAP:SPED). Projective test in assessment of high-risk youth. A measurement validation. *Student Dissertation Abstracts International, A: The Humanities and Social Sciences*, 61(7), 7920-A.

McCombs, D., Filipczak, J., Friedman R. M., & Wodarski, J. S. (1978). Long-term follow-up of behavior modification with high-risk adolescents. *Criminal Justice and Behavior*, 5(1), 21–34.

Meyer, R. G., & Smith., S. R. (1977). A crisis in group therapy. *American Psychologist*, 32(8), 638–643.

Mickle, J. (1963). Psychiatric home visits. *Archives of General Psychiatry*, 9, 379–383.

Moynihan, S. K. (1974). Home visits for family treatment. *Social Casework*, 55(10), 612–617.

Mrug, S., Hoza, B., & Gerdes, A. C. (2001). Children with attention-deficit/hyperactivity disorder: Peer relationships and peer-oriented interventions. In D. W. Nangle & C. A. Erdley (Eds.), *The role of friendship in psychological adjustment: New directions for child and adolescent development* (pp. 51–77). San Francisco, CA: Jossey-Bass.

Nickelson, D. W. (1995). The future of professional psychology in a changing health care marketplace: A conversation with Russ Newman. *Professional Psychology: Research and Practice*, 26(4), 366–370.

Reid, W. J. (1978). *The task centered system*. New York: Columbia University Press.

Reid, W. J., & Hanrahan, P. (1982). Recent evaluations of social work. Grounds for optimism. *Social Work*, 27(4), 328–340.

Richmond, M. E. (1971). *Social diagnosis*. New York: Russell Sage Foundation.

Roberts, C. S., Cox, C. E., Shannon, V. J., & Wells, N. L. (1994). A closer look at social support as a moderator of stress in breast cancer. *Health Social Work*, 19, 157–164.

Rose, S. D. (1977). *Group therapy: A behavioral approach*. Oxford, UK: Prentice-Hall.

Rubin, A. (1985). Practice effectiveness: More grounds for optimism. *Social Work*, 30(6), 469–476.

Ryan, W. (1971). *Blaming the victim*. New York: Vintage Books.

Sanderson, W. C., & Woody, S. (1995). Manuals for empirically supported treatments. *The Clinical Psychologist*, 48(4), 7–11.

Schulte D., Kunzel, R., Pepping, G., & Schulte-Bahrenberg, T. (1992). Tailor-made versus standardized therapy of phobic patients. *Advances in Behaviour Research and Therapy*, 14(2), 67–92.

Shadish, W. R., & Baldwin, S. A. (2003, October). Meta-analysis of MFT interventions. *Journal of Marital and Family Therapy*, 29(4), 547–570.

Shapiro, R. J. (1974, August). Therapist attitudes and premature termination in family and individual therapy. *Journal of Nervous and Mental Disease*, 159(2), 101–107.

Shealy, C. N. (1995). From Boys Town to Oliver Twist: Separating fact from fiction in welfare reform and out of-home placement of children and youth. *American Psychologist*, 50(8), 565–580.

Sheard, T., & Maguire, P. (1996, October). The effect of psychological interventions on anxiety and depression in oncology: Results of two meta-analyses. Paper presented at the Third World Congress of Psycho-Oncology, New York.

Shefler, G., Dasberg, H., & Ben Shakhar, G. (1995). A randomized controlled outcome and follow-up study of Mann's time-limited psychotherapy. *Journal of Consulting and Clinical Psychology*, 63(4), 585–593.

Stein, D. M., & Lambert, M. J. (1995). Graduate training in psychotherapy: Are therapy outcomes enhanced? *Journal of Consulting and Clinical Psychology*, 63(2), 182–196.

Stein, L. I., & Test, M. A. (1980). Alternative to mental hospital treatment: I. Conceptual model, treatment program, and clinical evaluation. *Archives of General Psychiatry*, 37(4), 392–397.

Stuart, R. B. (1974). *Trick or treatment*. Champaign, IL: Research Press.

Tapper, V. J. (1999). Psychotherapeutic trials specific to women with breast cancer: The state of science. *Journal of Psychosocial Oncology*, 17(3/4), 85–99.

Thomlison, R. J. (1984, Jan-Feb). Something works: Evidence from practice effectiveness studies. *Social Work*, 29(1), 51–56.

Thyer, B. A. (1995a). Constructivism and solipsism: Old wine in new bottles? *Social Work in Education*, 17, 63–64.

Thyer, B. A. (1995b). Effective psychosocial treatments for children and adolescents: A selected review. *Early Child Development and Care*, 106, 137–147.

Thyer, Bruce A. (2001, Winter). What is the role of theory in research on social work practice. *Journal of Social Work Education*, 37(1), 9–25, Social Services Abstracts.

Thyer, B. A., & Wodarski, J. S. (Eds.) (1998). *Handbook of empirical social work practice, Volume 1: Mental disorders*. New York: John Wiley & Sons.

Tyer, B. A., & Wodarski, J. S. (2007). *Social work in mental health: An evidence-based approach*. Hoboken, NJ: John Wiley & Sons.

Vaughn, M. G., & Howard, M. O. (2004, March). Integrated psychosocial and opioid-antagonist treatment for alcohol dependence: A systematic review of controlled evaluations. *Social Work Research*, 28(1), 41.

Westwood, M. J., Keats, P. A., & Wilensky, P. (2003). Therapeutic enactment: Integrating individual and group counseling models for change. *The Journal for Specialists in Group Work*, 28(2), 122–138.

Wilson, P. H. (1996). Prevention of recurrent depression. In P. Cotton & H. Jackson (Eds.), *Early intervention & prevention in mental health* (pp. 173–191). Carlton South, Victoria, Australia: Australian Psychological Society.

Witkin, S. L. (1991). Empirical clinical practice: A critical analysis. *Social Work*, 36(2), 158–163.

Wodarski, J. S. (1997). *Research methods for clinical social workers: Empirical practice*. New York: Springer Publishing Company.

Wodarski, J. S. (1980). Procedures for the maintenance and generalization of achieved behavioral change. *Journal of Sociology and Social Welfare*, 7(2), 298–311.

Wodarski, J. S., & Bagarozzi, D. (1979). *Behavioral social work*. New York: Human Sciences Press.

Wodarski, J. S., Feit, M. D., & Green, R. K. (1995, March). Graduate social work education: A review of two decades of empirical research and considerations for the future. *Social Service Review*, 69(1), 108–130.

Wodarski, J. S., Pippin, J. A., & Daniels, M. (1988). Effects of graduate social work education on personality, values, and interpersonal skills. *Journal of Social Work Education*, 24(3), 266–277.

Wodarski, J. S., & Wodarski, L. A. (1993). *Curriculums and practical aspects of implementation: Preventive health services for sdolescents*. Lanham, MD: University Press of America.

Yutrzenka, B. A. (1995). Making a case for training in ethnic and cultural diversity in increasing treatment efficacy. *Journal of Consulting and Clinical Psychology*, 63(2), 197–206.

Zemor, R., & Shepel, L. F. (1989). Effects of breast cancer and mastectomy on emotional support and adjustment. *Social Science and Medicine*, 28, 19–27.

6   Behavioral Health: Adolescent

Adler, L., & Kandel, D. B. (1981). Cross-cultural perspectives on developmental stages in adolescent drug use. *Journal of Studies on Alcohol*, 42(9), 701–715.

ADAMHA (Alcohol, Drug Abuse, and Mental Health Administration) (1991). *National drug control strategy: Budget summary*. Washington, DC: U.S. Government Printing Office.

Allensworth, D. D., & Kolbe, L. J. (1987). The comprehensive school health program: Exploring an expanded concept. *Journal of School Health*, 57(10), 311.

Alonso-Aperte, E., & Varela-Moreiras, G. (2000). Drugs-nutrient interactions: A potential problem during adolescence. *European Journal of Clinical Nutrition*, 54 (Suppl. 1), S69-S74.

American Academy of Pediatrics: Committee on Substance Abuse (1999). Marijuana: A continuing concern for pediatricians. *American Academy of Pediatrics*, 194(4), Pt. 1, 982–985.

American Medical Association (1996). *GAPS: A comprehensive approach to adolescent clinical preventive services*. Instructional video, 16 min. AA89:96–864:750:11/96. Chicago, IL: Department of Adolescent Health.

American Medical Association (1997). *Guidelines for adolescent preventive services (GAPS): Recommendations monograph*. Chicago, IL: American Medical Association, Department of Adolescent Health.

Andrews, J. A., Hops, H., Ary, D., Lichtenstein, E., & Tildesley, E. (1991). The construction, validation and use of a Guttman scale of adolescent substance use: An investigation of family relationship. *Journal of Drug Issues*, 21, 557–572.

Ary, D. V., Biglan, A., Glasgow, R., Zoref, L., Black, C., Ochs, L., et al. (1990). The efficacy of social-influence preventive programs vs. "standard care": Are new initiatives needed? *Journal of Behavioral Medicine*, 13, 281–296.

Asch, R. H., Smith, C. G., Siler-Khodt, T. M., & Pauterstem, C. J. (1981). Effects of delta-9-tetrahydrocannabinol during the follicular phase of the rhesus monkey. *Journal of Clinical Endocrinology Metabolism*, 52, 50–55.

Barnes, G. M., & Welte, J. W. (1986). Adolescent alcohol abuse: Sub-group differences and relationships to other problem behaviors. *Journal of Adolescent Research*, 1, 79–94.

Barone, C., Weissberg, R. P., Kasprow, W. J., Voyce, C. K., Arthur, M. W., & Shriver, T. P. (1995). Involvement in multiple problem behaviors of young urban adolescents. *Journal of Primary Prevention*, 15(3), 261–283.

Barry, C. M. (2006, July). Friends' influence on prosocial behavior: The role of motivational factors and friendship characteristics. *Developmental Psychology*, 42, 153–163.

Basen-Engquist, K., Edmundson, E. W., & Parcel, C. S. (1996). Structure of health and behavior among high school students. *Journal of Consulting and Clinical Psychology*, 64, 764–775.

Bauman, A., & Phongsavan, P. (1999). Epidemiology of substance use in adolescence: Prevalence, trends, and policy implications. *Drug and Alcohol Dependence*, 55(3), 187–207.

Beane, J. (1990). 100 years of "just say no" versus "just say know": Reevaluating drug education goals for the coming century. *Evaluation Review*, 22(2), 39.

Bell, R. M., Ellickson, P. L., & Harrison, E. R. (1993). Do prevention effects persist into high school? How Project ALERT did with ninth graders. *Preventive Medicine*, 22, 463–483.

Botvin, G. J. (1985). The life skills training program as a health promotion strategy: Theoretical issues and empirical findings. *Special Services in the Schools*, 1(3), 9–23.

Botvin, G. J., Baker, E., Botvin, E. M., Filazzola, A. D., & Millman, R. B. (1984a). Prevention of alcohol misuse through the development of personal and social competence: A pilot study. *Journal of Studies on Alcohol*, 45(6), 552–553.

Botvin, G. J., Baker, E., Dusenbury, L., Botvin, E. M., & Diaz, T. (1995). Long-term follow-up results of a randomized drug abuse prevention trial in a white middle class population. *JAMA*, 273, 1106–1112.

Botvin, G. J., Baker, E., Renick, N. L., Filazzola, A. D., & Botvin, E. M. (1984b). A cognitive-behavioral approach to substance abuse prevention. *Addictive Behaviors*, 9, 137–147.

Brener N. D., & Collins, J. L. (1998). Co-occurrence of health-risk behaviors among adolescents in the United States. *Journal of Adolescent Health*, 22, 209–213.

Brook, J. S., Brook, D. W., Gordon, A. S., Whiteman, M., & Cohen, P. (1990). The psychosocial etiology of adolescent drug use: A family interactional approach. *Genetic, Social, and General Psychological Monographs*, 116(2).

Brown, B. B. (1990). Peer groups and peer cultures. In S. S. Feldman & G. R. Elliot (Eds.), *At the threshold: The developing adolescent* (pp. 171–196). Cambridge, MA: Harvard University Press.

Bruner, A. B., & Fishman, M. (1998). Adolescent and illicit drug use. *Journal of the American Medical Association*, 280(7), 597–598.

Bruvold, W. H. (1993). A meta-analysis of adolescent smoking prevention programs. *American Journal of Public Health*, 83, 872–880.

Cabral, G. (1996). Effects of marijuana on the brain, endocrine system and immune system. In *Conference highlights: National Conference on Marijuana Use: Prevention, treatment and research* (pp. 21–24). Rockville, MD: National Institute on Drug Abuse, National Institutes of Health; NIH publication 96–4106.

Carboni, E., Acquas, E., Frau, R., & Di Chiara, G. (1989). Differential inhibitory effects of a 5-HT3 antagonist on drug-induced stimulation of dopamine release. *European Journal of Pharmacology*, 164(3), 515–519.

Carroll, M. D., Abraham, S., & Dresser, C. M. (1983). Dietary intake source data: United States 1976–1980. (Vital and Health Statistics, Series II, 231 USDHHS, PHS, NCHS, DHHS, Publication No. 83–1681). Washington, DC: National Center for Health Statistics.

CDC (2004). State specific prevalence of current cigarette smoking among adults—United States, 2003. *MMWR*, 53(44), 1035–1037.

Chaiken, M. R. (1993). The rise of crack and ice: Experiences in three locales. *Research in Brief*, NCJ 139559. Washington, DC: Government Printing Office.

Cohen, S. (1985). Marijuana and reproductive functions. *Drug Abuse and Alcohol News*, 13(1).

Cornelius, M. D., Taylor, P. M., Geva, D., & Day, N. L. (1995). Prenatal tobacco and marijuana use among adolescents: Effects on offspring gestational age, growth, and morphology. *Pediatrics*, 95, 738–743.

Cottrell, J. C., Sohn, S. S., & Vogel, W. H. (1973). Toxic effects of marijuana, tar on mouse skin. *Archives of Environmental Health*, 26, 277–278.

Denny, R. C., & Johnson, R. (1984). Nutrition, alcohol and drug abuse. *Proceedings of the Nutritional Society*, 43, 265–270.

Dishion, T. J., & Andrews, D. W. (1995). Preventing escalation in problem behaviors with high-risk young adolescents: Immediate and 1-year outcomes. *Journal of Consulting and Clinical Psychology*, 63(4), 538–548.

Donaldson, S. I., Graham, J. W., & Hansen, W. B.(1994). Testing the generalizability of intervening mechanism theories: Understanding the effects of adolescent drug use prevention interventions. *Journal of Behavioral Medicine*, 17(2), 195–216.

Donovan, J., & Jessor, R. (1985). Structure of problem behavior in adolescence and young adulthood. *Journal of Consulting and Clinical Psychology*, 53, 890–904.

Donovan, J., Jessor, R., & Costa, F. M. (1988). Syndrome of problem behavior in adolescence: A replication. *Journal of Consulting and Clinical Psychology*, 56, 762–765.

Driskell, J. A., Clark, A. J., & Moak, S. W. (1987). Longitudinal assessment of vitamin B-6 status in southern adolescent girls. *Journal of the American Dietetic Association*, 87, 307.

Dryfoos, J. G. (1991) *Adolescents at risk: Prevalence and prevention*. New York: Oxford University Press.

Dryfoos, J. G. (1990) *Adolescent at risk*. New York: Oxford University Press.

DuRant, R. H., Kahn, J., Beckford, P. H., & Woods, E. R. (1997a). The association of weapon carrying and fighting on school property and other health risk and problem behaviors among high school students. *Archives of Pediatrics & Adolescent Medicine*, 153(3), 286.

DuRant, R. H., Knight, J., & Goodman, E. (1997b). Factors associated with aggressive and delinquent behaviors among patients attending an adolescent medicine clinic. *Journal of Adolescent Health*, 21, 303–308.

DuRant, R. H., Smith, J. A., Kreiter, S. R., & Krowchuk, D. P. (1999). The relationship between early age of onset of initial substance use and engaging in multiple health risk behaviors among young adolescents. *Archives of Pediatrics & Adolescent Medicine*, 153(3), 286.

Eisen, M., Zellman, G. L., & McAlister, A. L. (1990). Evaluating the impact of a theory-based sexuality and contraceptive education program. *Family Planning Perspectives*, 22(6), 261–271.

Elixhauser, A. (1990). The costs of smoking and the cost-effectiveness of smoking-cessation programs. *Journal of Public Health Policy*, 11(2), 218–237.

Ellickson, P. L., Bell, R. M., & McGuigan, K. (1993). Preventing adolescent drug use: Long-term results of a junior high program. *American Journal of Public Health*, 83, 856–861.

Ellickson, P. L., Hays, R. D., & Bell, R. M. (1992). Stepping through the drug use sequence: Longitudinal scalogram of initiation and regular use. *Journal of Abnormal Psychology*, 101(3), 441–451.

Elliott, D. S., Huizinga, D., & Ageton, S. S. (1985). *Explaining delinquency and drug use*. Beverly Hills, CA: Sage Publications.

Escobedo, L. G., Reddy, M., & DuRant, R. H. (1997). Relationship of cigarette smoking to health risk and problem behaviors among US adolescents. *Archives of Pediatric Adolescent Medicine*, 151, 66–71.

Evans, R. I., Rozelle, R. M., Mittelmark, M., Hansen, W. B., Bane, A. L., & Havis, J. (1978). Deterring the onset of smoking in children: Knowledge of immediate physiological effects and coping with peer pressure, media pressure, and parents modeling. *Journal of Applied Social Psychology*, 8(2), 126–135.

Everett, S. A., Kann, L., & McReynolds, L. (1997). The youth risk behavior surveillance system: Policy and program application. *Journal of School Health*, 67, 333–335.

Fagan, J., Weis, J. G., & Cheng, Y. T. (1990). Delinquency and substance use among inner-city students. *Journal of Drug Issues*, 20, 351–402.

Falco, M. (1992). *The making of a drug free America*. New York: Times Books.

Farquhar, J. W., Fortman, S. D., Flora., J. A., Taylor, C. B., Haskell, W. L., Williams, P. T. et al. (1990). Effects of community wide education on cardiovascular disease risk factors: The Stanford five-city project. *JAMA*, 264, 359–365.

Farrell, A. D., Danish, S. J., & Howard, C. W. (1992). Relationship between drug use and other problem behaviors in urban adolescents. *Journal of Consulting and Clinical Psychology*, 60(5), 705–712.

Farrow, J. A., Rees, J. M., & Worthington-Roberts, B. S. (1987). Health, developmental, and nutritional status of adolescent alcohol and marijuana users. *Pediatrics*, 79, 218.

Fisher, M., Schneider, M., Pegler, C., & Napolitano, B. (1991). Eating attitudes, health risk behaviors, self-esteem, and anxiety among females in a suburban high school. *Journal of Adolescent Health*, 12, 377–384.

Foltin, R. W., Brady, J. V., & Fischman, M. W. (1986). Behavioral analysis of marijuana effects on food intake in humans. *Pharmacology and Bio-behavioral Behavior*, 25, 277.

Forster, J. L., & Wolfson, M. (1998, May). Youth access to tobacco: Policies and politics. *Annual Review of Public Health*, 19, 203–235.

Frank, G. (1998). Nutrition for teens. In A. Henderson, S. Champlin, & W. Evashwick (Eds.), *Promoting teen health: Linking schools, health organizations, and community*. Thousand Oaks, CA: Sage Publications.

French, J. R. P. (1956). A formal theory of social power. *Psychological Review*, 63, 181–194.

French, J. R. P., & Raven, B. H. (1959). The bases of social power. In D. Cartwright (Ed.), *Studies in social power* (pp. 150–167). Ann Arbor, MI: Institute for Social Research, University of Michigan.

Fried, P. A. (1995). The Ottawa prenatal prospective study (OPPS): Methodological issues and findings—it's easy to throw the baby out with the bath water. *Life Sciences*, 56, 2159–2168.

Fulgoni, V. L., & Mackey, M. A. (1991). Total dietary fiber in children's diets. In C. L. Williams & E. L. Wynder (Eds.), *Hyperlipidemia and the development of artheroschlerosis*. Annual of the New York Academy of Science, 623, 369–379.

Gans, J. E., Alexander, B., Chu, R. C., & Elster, A. B. (1995). The cost of comprehensive preventive medical services for adolescents. *Archives of Pediatric and Adolescent Medicine*, 149, 1226–1234.

Garmezy, N. (1991). Resiliency and vulnerability to adverse developmental outcomes associated with poverty. *American Behavioral Scientist*, 34, 416–430.

Gillmore, M. R., Hawkings, D. J., Catalona, R. F., Day, L. E., Moore, M., & Abott, R. (1991). Structure of problem behaviors in preadolescence. *Journal of Consulting and Clinical Psychology*, 59, 499–506.

Giugliano, D. (1984). Morphine, opioid, peptides, and pancreatic islet of function. *Diabetes Care*, 7, 92.

Golub, A. L., & Johnson, B. D. (1996). The crack epidemic: Empirical findings support a hypothesized diffusion of innovation process. *Socio-Economic Planning Sciences*, 30(3), 221–223.

Golub, A. L., & Johnson, B. D. (1997). Crack's decline: Some surprises across U. S. cities. *Research in brief*, NCJ 165707. Washington, DC: Government Printing Office.

Graham, J. W., Collins, L. M., Wugalter, S. E., Chung, N. K., & Hansen, W. B. (1991a). Modeling transitions in latent stage-sequential processes: A substance use prevention example. *Journal of Consulting and Clinical Psychology*, 59, 48–57.

Graham, J. W., Marks, G., & Hansen, W. B. (1991b). Social influence processes affecting adolescent substance use. *Journal of Applied Psychology*, 76(2), 291–298.

Greenberg, I., Kuehnle, J., Mendelson, J. H., & Bernstein, J. G. (1976). Effects of marijuana use an body weight and caloric intake in humans. *Psychopharmacology*, 49, 79.

Grimley, D. M., & Lee, P. A. (1997). Condom and other contraceptive use among a random sample of female adolescents: A snapshot in time. *Adolescence*, 32(128), 771–779.

Gross, H. M., Elbert, H., Faden, V. B., Goldberg, S. C., Kaye, W. H., Caine, E. D., et al. (1983). A double-blind trial of delta-9-tetrahydrocannabinol on primary anorexia nervosa. *Journal of Clinical Psychopharmacology*, 3, 165.

Grunbaum, J. A., Kann, L., Kinchen, S. A., Ross J. G., Gowda, V. R., Collins, J. L., et al. (2000). Youth risk behavior surveillance national alternative high school youth risk behavior survey: United States, 1998. *Journal of School Health*, 70(1), 5.

Grunberg, N. E. (1982). The effect of nicotine and cigarette smoking on food consumption and taste preferences. *Addictive Behavior*, 7, 317.

Hamid, A. (1992). The development cycle of a drug epidemic: The cocaine smoking epidemic of 1981–1991. *Journal of Psychoactive Drugs*, 24(4), 337–348.

Hansen, W. B. (1992). School-based substance abuse prevention: A review of the state of the art in curriculum, 1980–1998. *Health Education Research and Theory Practice*, 7, 403–430.

Harris, L. (1988). *An evaluation of comprehensive health education in American public schools.* New York: Metropolitan Life Foundation.

Hawkins, J. D., Catalano, R. F., Kosterman, R., Abbott, R., & Hill, K. G. (1999). Preventing adolescent health-risk behaviors by strengthening protection during childhood. *Archives of Pediatric and Adolescent Medicine*, 153, 226–234.

Hofferth, S. L., & Miller, B. C. (1989). An overview of adolescent pregnancy prevention programs and their evaluations. In J. J. Card (Ed.), *Evaluating programs aimed at preventing teenage pregnancies* (pp. 25–40). Palo Alto, CA: Sociometrics Corporation, Data Archive on Adolescent Pregnancy and Pregnancy Prevention.

Hollister, L. E. (1971). Hunger and appetite after single doses of marihuana, alcohol, and dextroamphetamine. *Clinical Pharmacology and Therapeutics,* 12, 44–99.

Howard, M. (1992). Delaying the start of intercourse among adolescents. *Adolescent Medicine: State of the Art Reviews,* 3, 181–193.

Howard, M., & McCabe, J. A. (1992). An information and skills approach for younger teens: Postponing sexual involvement program. In B. C. Miller, J. J. Card, R. L., Paikoff, & J. L. Peterson (Eds.), *Preventing adolescent pregnancy: Model programs and evaluations* (pp. 83–109). Newbury Park, CA: Sage Publications.

Hoyumpa, A. M., & Schenker, S. (1982). Major drug interactions: Effects of liver disease, alcohol, and malnutrition. *Annals Review of Medicine,* 33, 113–149.

Irwin, C. E. (1989). Risk taking behaviors in the adolescent patient: Are they impulsive? *Pediatric Annuals,* 18, 122–133.

Irwin, C. E., & Ryan, S. A. (1989). Problem behavior of adolescents. *Pediatrics in Review,* 10, 235–246.

Jainchill, N., Yagelka, J., Hawke, J., & DeLeon, G. (1999). Adolescent admissions to residential drug treatment: HIV risk behaviors pre-and post-treatment. *Psychology of Addictive Behaviors,* 13(3), 163–173.

James, W. H., Moore, D. D., & Gregersen, M. M. (1996). Early prevention of alcohol and other drug use among adolescents. *Journal of Drug Education,* 26(2), 131–142.

Jessor, R. (1987) Problem-behavior theory, psychosocial development and adolescent problem drinking. *British Journal of Addiction,* 82, 331–342.

Jessor, R. (1991). Risk behavior in adolescence: A psychological framework for understanding and action. *Journal of Adolescent Health,* 12, 597–605.

Jessor, R. (1992). Risk behavior in adolescence: A psychosocial framework for understanding and action. *Journal of Adolescent Health,* 21, 597–605.

Jessor, R., Donovan, J. E., & Costa, F. M. (1991). *Beyond adolescence: Problem behavior and young adult development.* New York: Cambridge University Press.

Jessor, R., & Jessor, S. L. (1977). *Problem behavior and psychological development.* San Diego, CA: Academic Press.

Johnston, L. D., O'Malley, P. M., & Bachman, J. G. (1998). *National Survey Results on drug use from the monitoring the future study, 1975–1997: Volume 1: Secondary school students.* NIH Publication No. 98–4345. Rockville, MD: National Institute on Drug Abuse.

Johnston, L. D., O'Malley, P. M., & Bachman, J. G. (1995). *National Survey Results on drug use from the monitoring the future study, 1975–1994. Volume 1: Secondary school students.* NIH Publication No. 95–4026, Rockville, MD: National Institute on Drug Abuse.

Johnston, L. D., O'Malley, P. M., & Bachman, J. G. (1996). *National Survey Results on drug use from the monitoring the future study 1975–1995. Volume 1: Secondary school students.* NIH Publication No. 96–4139. Rockville, MD: National Institute on Druge Abuse.

Johnston, L. D., O'Malley, P. M., Bauchman, J. G., & Schulenberg, J. E. (2005). *Monitoring the future national results on adolescent drug use: Overview of key findings, 2004.* NIH Publication No. 05–5726, Bethesda, MD: National Institute on Drug Abuse.

Jonas, J. M., Gold, M. S., Sweeney, D., & Pattash, A. L. C. (1987). Eating disorders and cocaine abuse: A survey of 259 cocaine abusers. *Journal of Clinical Psychiatry,* 48, 47.

Jorgensen, S. R. (1991). Project taking charge: An evaluation of an adolescent pregnancy prevention program. *Family Relations*, 40, 373–380.

Kandel, D. (1975). Stages in adolescent involvement in drug use. *Science*, 190, 912–914.

Kandel, D., & Davies M. (1991). Cocaine use in a national sample of U.S. youth (NLSY): Ethnic patterns, progression, and predictors. In S. Schober & C. Schade (Eds.), *The epidemiology of cocaine use and abuse (NIDA Research Monograph 110)* (pp. 151–188). Washington, DC: U.S. Department of Health and Human Services.

Kandel, D., & Yamaguchi, K. (1993). From beer to crack: Developmental patterns of drug involvement. *American Journal of Public Health*, 83, 851–855.

Kandel, D., Yamaguchi, K., & Chen, K. (1992). Stages of progression in drug involvement from adolescence to adulthood: Further evidence for the gateway theory. *Journal of Studies on Alcohol*, 53, 447–457.

Kann, L., Kinchen, S. A., Williams, B. I., Ross, J. G., Lowry, R., Hill, C. V. et al. (1998). Youth risk behavior surveillance—United States, 1997. *Division of Adolescent and School Health, National Center for Chronic Disease Prevention and Health Promotion*, 47 (SS-3), 1–89.

Kann, L., Kolbe, L. J., & Collins, J. L. (Eds.) (1993). Measuring the health behavior of adolescents: The youth risk behavior surveillance system. *Public Health Reports*, 108 (Suppl. 1), 1–67.

Kann, L., Warren, C. W., Harris, W. A., Collins, J. L., Williams, B. I., Ross, J. G., et al. (1996). Youth risk behavior surveillance: United States, *MMWR*, 45(SS-4), 1–84.

Kaplan, H. I., & Saddock, B. J. (1991). *Synopsis of psychiatry: Behavioral sciences clinical psychiatry* (6th ed.). Baltimore, MD: Williams & Wilkins.

Kersting, K. (2005, September). Study indicates mental illness toll on youth, delays in treatment. *Monitor on Psychology*, 15.

Kelman, H. C. (1958). Compliance, identification, and internalization: Three processes of attitude change. *Journal of Conflict Resolution*, 2, 51–60.

Kelman, H. C. (1961). Process of opinion change. *Public Opinion Quarterly*, 25, 57–78.

Kim, S., Crutchfield, C., Williams, C., & Helper, N. (1998). Toward a new paradigm in substance abuse and other problem prevention for youth: Youth development and empowerment approach. *Journal of Drug Education*, 28(1), 1–17.

Kirby, D., Short, L., Collins, J., Rugg, D., Kolbe, L., Howard M., et al. (1994). School-based programs to reduce sexual risk behaviors: A review of effectiveness. *Public Health Reports*, 109(3), 339–360.

Klitzner, M. D., Fisher, D., Moskowitz, J., Stewart, K., & Gilbert, S. (1991). Report to the Robert Wood Johnson Foundation on "Strategies to Prevent the Onset and Use of Addictive and Abusable Substances among Children and Early Adolescents." Bethesda, MD: Pacific Institute for Research and Evaluation.

Kokotailo, P. (1995). Physical health problems associated with adolescent substance abuse. *National Institute of Drug Abuse Research Monographs*, 156, 112–129.

Kokotailo, P., & Adger, H. (1991). Substance use by pregnant adolescents. *Clinics in Perinatology*, 18, 125–138.

Kolbe, L. J., Kann, L., & Collins, J. L. (1993). Overview of the youth risk behavior surveillance system. *Public Health Reports*, 108 (Suppl. 1), 2–10.

Kropp, B. Y., & Halpern-Felsher, B. L. (2004, October). Adolescents' beliefs about the risks involved in smoking "light" cigarettes. From the Division of Adolescent

Medicine, Department of Pediatrics, University of California, San Francisco, California. *Pediatrics*, 114(4), e445-e451 (doi:10.1542/peds. 2004–0893).

Lester, B. M., & Dreher, M. (1989). Effects of marijuana use during pregnancy on newborn cry. *Child Development*, 60(4), 765–771.

Levenberg, P. B., & Elster, A. B. (1995a). *Guidelines for adolescent preventive services (GAPS): Implementation and resource manual*. Chicago, IL: American Medical Association, Department of Adolescent Health.

Levenberg, P. B., & Elster, A. B. (1995b). *Guidelines for adolescent preventive services (GAPS): Clinical evaluation and management handbook*. Chicago, IL: American Medical Association, Department of Adolescent Health.

Levy, D. A., Collins, B. E., & Nail, P. R. (1998). A new model of interpersonal influence characteristics. *Journal of Social Behavior and Personality*, 13(4), 715–733.

Levy, S. J., & Pierce, J. P. (1990). Predictors of marijuana use and take among teenagers in Sydney, Australia. *International Journal of Addictions*, 25, 1179–1193.

Lopez, M. C., Huang, D. S., Chen, G. J., & Watson, R. R. (1991). Splencyote subsets in normal and protein malnourished mice after long-term exposure to cocaine and morphine. *Life Sciences*, 17, 1253–1262.

Luthar, S., & Ziegler, E. (1991). Vulnerability and competence: A review of research on resilience in children. *American Journal of Orthopsychiatry*, 61, 6–22.

Marquis, D. K., & Wagner, S. (1997). *Guidelines for adolescent preventive services (GAPS): Implementation training workbook* (3rd ed.), USA: American Medical Association.

Maternal and Child Health Bureau, Public Health Service (1995). *Child health USA '94*. Washington, DC: U.S. Department of Health and Human Services. DHHS Publication No. HRSA-MCH-95-1.

McCaul, K. D., & Glasgow, R. E. (1985). Preventing adolescent smoking: What have we learned about treatment construct validity? *Health Psychology*, 4, 361–387.

McDowell, U., & Futris, T. G. (2002). *Adolescents at risk: Illicit drug use*. Ohio State University Extension, FLM-FS-15–02, Fact Sheet, Family Life Month Packet 2002.

McGee. L., & Newcomb, M. D. (1992). General deviance syndrome: Expanded hierarchical evaluations at four ages from early adolescence to adulthood. *Journal of Consulting and Clinical Psychology*, 60(5), 766–776.

Merrill, J. C., Kleber, H. D., Shwartz, M., Liu, H., & Lewis, S. R. (1999). Cigarettes, alcohol, marijuana, other risk behaviors, and American youth. *Drug and Alcohol Dependence*, 56, 205–212.

Millstein, S. G., & Litt, I. F. (1990). Adolescent health. In S. S. Feldman & G. R. Elliot (Eds.), *At the threshold: The developing adolescent* (pp. 431–456). Cambridge, MA: Harvard University Press.

Mitchell, C. M., & Beals, J. (1997). The structure of problem and positive behavior among American Indian adolescents: Gender and community differences. *American Journal of Community Psychology*, 25(3), 257–288.

Moberg, D. P., & Piper, D. L. (1998). The healthy for life project: Sexual risk behavior outcomes. *AIDS Education and Preventing*, 10(20), 128–148.

Mohs, M. E., Watson, R. R., & Leonard-Green, T. (1990). Nutritional effects of marijuana, heroin, cocaine, and nicotine. *Journal of the American Dietetic Association*, 90, 1261–1267.

Mott, F. L., & Haurin, R. J. (1988). Linkages between sexual activity and alcohol and drug use among American adolescents. *Family Planning Perspectives*, 20, 128–136.

NCHS (National Center for Health Statistics) (1992). Trends in pregnancies and pregnancy rates, United States, 1980–1988. *Monthly Vital Statistics Report*, 41(6), 1–7.

NIDA (National Institute on Drug Abuse) (1980). Marijuana and Health. Eighth annual report to the U.S. Congress from the Secretary of Health and Human Services, 1980. Washington, DC: U.S. Government Printing Office.

National Organization for the Reform of Marijuana Laws (NORML) (2002). Marijuana not a gateway to hard drug use, rand study says conclusions raise serious doubts regarding the legitimacy of U.S. drug policy. Retrieved April 18, 2005, from http://www.norml.org/index.cfm?Group_ID=5490.

Nemark-Sztainer, D., Story, M., French, S. Cassto, N. Jacobs, D. R., & Resnick, M. D. (1996). Patterns of health-compromising behaviors among Minnesota adolescents: Sociodemographic variations. *American Journal of Public Health*, 86(11), 1599–1606.

Newcomb, M. D. (1995). Identifying high-risk youth: Prevalence and patterns of adolescent drug abuse. In E. Radert & D. Czechowicz (Eds.), *Adolescent drug abuse: Clinical assessment and therapeutic interventions NIDA research monograph (156)* (pp. 7–38). Rockville, MD: Department of Health and Human Services.

Newcomb, M. D., & Bentler, P. M. (1986). Substance use and ethnicity: Differential impact of peer and adult models. *Journal of Psychology*, 120, 83–95.

Newcomb, M. D., & Bentler, P. M. (1988). *Consequences of adolescent drug use*. Beverly Hills, CA: Sage Publications.

Newcomb, M. D., McCarthy, W. J., & Bentler, P. M. (1989). Cigarette smoking, academic lifestyle, and social impact efficacy: An eight-year study from early adolescence to young adulthood. *Journal of Applied Social Psychology*, 19, 251–281.

OTA (Office of Technology Assessment) (1991). *Adolescent health—Volume II: Background and the effectiveness of selected prevention and treatment services*, Report No. OTA-H-466. Washington, DC: U.S. Government Printing Office.

Olsen, J., Weed, S., Daly, D., & Jensen, L. (1992). The effects of abstinence sex education programs on virgin versus non-virgin students. *Journal of Research and Development in Education*, 25(2), 69–75.

Orleans, C. T., & Slade, J. (1993). *Nicotine addiction principles and management*. New York: Oxford University Press.

Pickoff-White, L. (2006, June 15). Many risky behaviors down among teenagers. *Science in the Headlines*. Retrieved July 6, 2006, from http://www.national academies.org/headlines/20060615.html.

Prince, F. (1995). The relative effectiveness of a peer-led and adult-led smoking intervention program. *Adolescence*, 30(117), 187–194.

Rabkin, S. (1984). Relationship between weight change and the reduction of cessation of cigarette smoking. *International Journal of Obesity*, 8, 665.

Raven, B. H. (1965). Social influence and power. In B. H. Raven & I. Z. Rubin (Eds.), *Social psychology* (2nd ed., pp. 399–443). New York: Holt, Rinehart & Winston.

Reed, J. L., & Ghodse, A. H. (1973). Oral glucose tolerance and hormonal response in heroin-dependent males. *British Medical Journal*, 2, 582.

Resikow, K., & Botvin, G. (1993). School-based substance use prevention programs: Why do effects decay? *Preventive Medicine*, 22, 484–490.

Resnick, M. D., Bearman, P. S., Blum, R. W., Bauman, K. E., Harris, K. M., Jones, J., et al. (1997). Protecting adolescents from harm: Findings from the national longitudinal study on adolescent health. *JAMA*, 278, 823–832.

Rhoads, K. (2002). An introduction to social influence. Retrieved April 18, 2005, from http://www.workingpsychology.com/intro.html.

Riggs, S., & Cheng, T. (1988). Adolescents' willingness to use a school-based clinic in view of expressed health concerns. *Journal of Adolescent Health*, 9, 208–213.

Rigotti, N. A. (2000). A 36-year-old woman who smokes cigarettes. *JAMA*, 284(6), 741–749.

Rigotti, N. A., Arnsten, J. H., McKool, K. M., Wood-Reid, K. M., Pasternak, R. C., & Singer, D. E. (1997). Efficacy of a smoking cessation program for hospital patients. *Archives of Internal Medicine*, 157(22). Retrieved from http://archinte. ama-assn.org/cigi/content/abstract/157/22/2653.

Robins, L. N., & Przybeck, T. R. (1985). Age of onset of drug use as a factor in drug and other disorders. In C. L. Jones & R. J. Batjes (Eds.), *Etiology of drug abuse: Implications for prevention* (Research Monograph No. 56, pp. 178–193). Rockville, MD: National Institute on Drug Abuse.

Robinson, T. N., Killen, J. Dl., Taylor, C. B., Telch, M. J., Bryson S. W., Saylor, K. E., et al. (1987). Perspectives on adolescent substance use: A defined population study. *JAMA*, 258(15), 2072–2076.

Roosa, M. W., & Christopher, F. S. (1990). Evaluation of an abstinence-only adolescent pregnancy prevention program: A replication. *Family Relations*, 39, 363–367.

Rosenbaum, E., & Kandel, D. B. (1990). Early onset of adolescent sexual behavior and drug involvement. *Journal of Marriage and the Family*, 52, 783–798.

Rosenbaum, M. (1996). *Kids, drugs, and drug education: A harm reduction approach*. San Francisco, CA: National Council on Crime and Delinquency.

Rosenbaum, M. (1998). "Just say know" to teenagers and marijuana. *Journal of Psychoactive Drugs*, 30(2), 197–203.

Rutter, M. (1993). Resilience: Some conceptual considerations. *Journal of Adolescent Health*, 14, 626–639.

Sarigiani, P. A., Ryan, L., & Petersen, A. C. (1999). Prevention of high risk-risk behaviors in adolescent women. *Journal of Adolescent Health*, 20, 373–383.

Schinke, S. P. (1982). A school-based model for teenage pregnancy prevention. *Social Work Education*, 4, 32–42.

Schinke, S. P., Botvin, G. J., Trimble, J. E., Orlandi, M. A., Gilchrist, L. D., & Locklear, V. S. (1988). Preventing substance abuse among American-Indian adolescents: A bicultural competence skills approach. *Journal of Counseling Psychology*, 35, 87–90.

Seffrin, J. R., & Bailey, W. J. (1985). Approaches to adolescent smoking cessation and education. *Special Services in the Schools*, 1(3), 25–38.

Shedler, J., & Block, J. (1990). Adolescent drug use and psychological health: A longitudinal inquiry. *American Psychologist*, 45, 612–630.

Shope, J. T., Copeland, L. A., Kamp, M. E., & Lang, S. W. (1998). Effectiveness of a school-based substance abuse prevention program. *Journal of Drug Education*, 26(4), 323–337.

Shrier, L. A., Emans, J., Woods, E. R., & DuRant, R. H. (1997). The association of sexual risk behaviors and problem drug behaviors in high school students. *Journal of Adolescent Health*, 20(5), 377–383.

Simon, T. R., Richardson, J. L., Dent. C. W., Chow, C. P., & Flay, B. R. (1998). Prospective psychosocial, interpersonal, and behavioral predictors of handgun carrying among adolescents. *American Journal of Public Health*, 88, 960–963.

Slavin, R., Karwelt, N. L., & Madden, N. A. (1990). *Effective programs for students at risk.* Boston, MA: Allyn & Bacon.

Spingarn, R. W., & DuRant, R. H. (1996). Male adolescents who cause pregnancy, associated health risk and problem behaviors. *Pediatrics,* 98, 262–268.

Stephenson, C. (1991). *Teaching 10 to 14 year olds.* White Plains, NY: Longman.

Stimmel, B. (1996). *Drug abuse and social policy in America: The war that must be won.* New York: Haworth Press.

Story, M. (1984). Nutritional needs and concerns of chronically ill adolescents. In R. W. Burn (Ed.), *The chronically ill and disabled adolescent.* New York: Grune & Stratton.

Story, M., & VanZyl York, P. (1987). Nutritional status of Native American adolescent substance users. *Journal of the American Dietetic Association,* 87, 1680.

Strunin, L., & Hingson, R. (1992). Alcohol, drugs, and adolescent sexual behavior. *International Journal of Addictions,* 27, 129–146.

Tanford, S., & Penrod, S. (1984). Social influence model: A formal integration of research on majority and minority influence processes. *Psychological Bulletin,* 95, 189–225.

Tobler, N. S. (1992). Drug prevention programs can work: Research findings. *Journal of Addictive Diseases,* 11, 1–28.

Turner, K. M., Gordon, J., & Young, R. (2004). Cigarette access and pupil smoking rates: A circular relationship. *Health Promotion International,* 19, 428–436.

U.S. Department of Education. Office of Safe and Drug-Free Schools. Retrieved April 22, 2005, from http://www.ed.gov/about/offices/list/odsfs/programs.html.

U.S. Department of Health and Human Services (1997). *Alcohol and health: Ninth special report to the U.S. Congress.* Washington, DC: Department of Health and Human Services.

U. S. General Accounting Office (1993). *Drug use among youth: No simple answers to guide prevention.* (Report to the Chairman, Subcommittee on Children, Family, Drugs, and Alcoholism, Committee on Labor and Human Resources, U. S. Senate.) Washington, DC: U.S. General Accounting Office (General Accounting Office report GAO/HRD-94-24).

U.S. General Accounting Office (1997). *Substance abuse and violence prevention: Multiple programs raise questions of efficiency and effectiveness.* Washington, DC: U.S. General Accounting Office.

U.S. Public Health Service (1991). *Healthy people 2000: National health promotion and disease prevention objectives.* Washington, DC: U.S. Government Printing Offices, DHHS Publication No. (PHS) 91–50212.

UMNIS (University of Michigan News and Information Services) (1997). *Monitoring the future study* [News Release]. Ann Arbor, MI: University of Michigan News and Information Services.

Warren, C. W., Kann, L., Small, M. S., Santelli, J. S., Collins, J. S., & Kolbe, L. J. (1997). Age of initiating selected health-risk behaviors among high school students in the United States. *Journal of Adolescent Health,* 21, 224–231.

Watson, R. R. (1988). Ethanol, immunomodulation and cancer. *Proceedings of Food and Nutrition Science,* 189–209.

Watson, R. R. (1992). LP-BM5, a murine model of acquired immunodeficiency syndrome: Role of cocaine, morphine, alcohol and carotenoids in nutritional immunomodulation. *Journal of Nutrition,* 122, 744–748.

Watson, R. R., & Mohs, M. E. (1989). Effects of morphine, cocaine, and heroin on nutrition. *Proceedings in Clinical Biological Research,* 325, 413–418.

Watson, R. R., & Mohs, M. E. (1990). Effects of morphine, cocaine and heroin. *Alcohol, Immunomodulation, and AIDS*, 413–418.

Weil, A. T. (1970). Adverse reactions to marijuana. Classification and suggested treatment. *New England Journal of Medicine*, 282(18), 997–1000.

Welte, J. W., & Barnes, G. M. (1985). Alcohol: The gateway to other drug use among secondary-school students. *Journal of Youth and Adolescence*, 14(6), 487–498.

Wetter, D. W., Fiore, M. C., Gritz, E. R., Lando, H. A., Stitzer, M. L., Haselblad, V., et al. (1998). The agency for health care policy and research smoking cessation clinical practice guideline. Findings and implications for psychologists. *American Psychologist*, 53(6), 657–669.

Witte, E. H. (1987). Behavior in group situations: An integrate model. *European Journal of Social Psychology*, 17, 403–429.

Witte, E. H. (1990). Social influence: A discussion and integration of recent models into a general group situation theory. *European Journal of Social Psychology*, 20, 3–27.

Wodarski, J. S. (1988). Teams—games—tournaments: Teaching adolescents about alcohol and driving. *Journal of Alcohol and Drug Education*, 33(3), 46–57.

Wodarski, J. S. (1990). Adolescent substance abuse: Practice implications. *Adolescence*, 25(99), 667–688.

Wodarski, J. S. (1992–1993). Teaching adolescents about alcohol and driving: An empirically validated program for social workers. *Research on Social Work Practice*, 4(1), 28–39.

Wodarski, J. S., & Feit, M. D. (1995). *Adolescent substance abuse: An empirically based group preventive health paradigm*. New York: Haworth Press.

Wodarski, L. A., & Wodarski, J. S. (1995). *Adolescent sexuality: A peer/family curriculum*. Springfield, IL: Charles C. Thomas.

Wood, P. B., Cochran, J. K., Pfefferbau, B., & Arneklev, B. J. (1995). Sensation-seeking and delinquent substance use: An extension of learning theory. *Journal of Drug Issues*, 25(1), 173–193.

Woods, E. R., Lin, V. G., Middleman, A., Beckford, P., Chase, L., & DuRant, R. H. (1997). The association of suicide attempts with other risks behaviors in adolescents in Massachusetts. *Pediatrics*, 99, 791–796.

Worchel, S., Copper J., & Goethals, G. R. (1988). *Understanding social psychology* (4th ed.). Chicago, IL: Dorsey Press.

Wozniak, K. M., Pert A., & Linnoila, M. (1990). Antagonism of 5-HT3 receptors attenuates the effects of ethanol on extracellular dopamine. *European Journal of Pharmacology*, 187(2), 287–289.

Yamaguchi, K., & Kandel, D. B. (1984). Patterns of drug use from adolescence to young adulthood: III. Predictors of progression. *American Journal of Public Health*, 74(7), 673–681.

Yu, J., & Williford, W. R. (1992). The age of alcohol onset and alcohol, cigarette, and marijuana use patterns: An analysis of drug use progression of young adults in New York State. *International Journal of the Addictions*, 27(11), 1313–1323.

Yu, J., & Williford, W. R. (1994). Alcohol, other drugs and criminality: A structural analysis. *American Journal of Drug and Alcohol Abuse*, 20(3), 373–393.

7 Adult Behavioral Health

Abramson, E. E. (1973, November). A review of behavioral approaches to weight control. *Behaviour Research and Therapy*, 11(4), 547–556.

Abramson, E. E. (1977). Behavioral approaches to weight control. *Behavior Research and Therapy*, 11, 547–566.

Agras, W. S., Schneider, J. A., Arnow, B., & Raeburn, S. D. (1989). Cognitive behavioral and response treatments for bulimia nervosa. *Journal of Consulting and Clinical Psychology*, 51(5), 634–636.

AGS (American Geriatric Society Panel on Chronic Pain in Older Persons) (1998). The management of chronic pain in older persons. *Journal of the American Geriatric Society*, 46(5), 635–651.

Allen, K. D., & Shriver, M. D. (1998). Role of parent-mediated pain behavior management strategies in biofeedback treatment of childhood migraines. *Behavior Therapy*, 29(3), 477–490.

Andersen, R. E., Franckowiak, S. C., Snyder, J., Bartlett, S. J., & Fontaine, K. R. (1998). Can inexpensive signs encourage the use of stairs? Results from a community intervention. *Annals of Internal Medicine*, 129, 363–369.

Andrasik, F., & Holroyd, K. A. (1983). Specific and nonspecific effects of biofeedback treatment of tension headache: Three year follow up. *Journal of Consulting and Clinical Psychology*, 51(4), 634–636.

Andres, R. (1980). Effect of obesity on total mortality. *International Journal of Obesity*, 4(4), 381–386.

Arena, J. G., Bruno, G. M., & Brucks, A. G. (1997). Chronic tension headache: The use of EMG biofeedback for the treatment of chronic tension headache. *Electromyography: Applications in chronic pain, physical medicine & rehabilitation*. Retrieved April 03, 2005, from http://www.bfe.org/protocol/pro08eng.html.

Arnold, E. (1997). The stress connection: Women and coronary heart disease. *Critical Care Nursing Clinics of North America*, 9(4), 565–575.

Baldwin, J. D., & Baldwin, J. J. (1986). *Behavioral principles in everyday* (2nd ed.). Englewood Cliffs, NJ: Prentice-Hall.

Bandura, A. (1969). *Principles of behavior modification*. New York: Holt, Rinehart & Winston.

Bandura, A. (1977). *Social learning theory*. Englewood Cliffs, NJ: Prentice-Hall.

Baranowski, T., Perry, C. L., & Parcel, G. S. (1997). How individuals, environments, and health behavior interact—social cognitive theory. In K. Glanz, F. M. Lewis, and B. Rimer (Eds.), *Health behavior and health education. Theory, research, and practice* (2nd ed., pp. 246–279). San Francisco, CA: Jossey-Bass.

Barendregt, J. J., Bonneux, L., & van der Maas, P. J. (1997). The health care costs of smoking. *The New England Journal of Medicine*, 337(15), 1052–1057.

Beach, L. R., Townes, B. O., Campbell, F. L., & Keating, G. W. (1976). Developing and testing a decision aid for birth planning decisions. *Organizational Behavioral and Human Performance*, 24, 19–28.

Berkman, B., Bonnander, E., Kemler, B., Marcus, L., Isaacson-Rubinger, M. J., Rutchick, I., et al. (1989). Social work and health care: A review of the literature. *Health and Social Work*, 14(3), 222–223.

Bjorntorp, P. (1978). Physical training in the treatment of obesity. *International Journal of Obesity*, 2(2), 149–156.

Blamey, A., Mutrie, N., & Aitchison, T. (1995). Health promotion by encouraged use of stairs. *British Medical Journal*, 311, 289–290.

Blanchard, E., & Andrasik, F. (1982, December). Psychological assessment and treatment of headache: Recent developments and emerging issues. *Journal of Consulting and Clinical Psychology*, 50(6), 859–879.

Blanchard, E. B., Andrasik, F., & Silver, B. V. (1980). Biofeedback and relaxation in the treatment of tension headaches: A reply to Belar. *Journal of Behavioral Medicine*, 3(3), 227–232.

Blanchard, E., Gordon, M., Wittrock, D., McCaffrey, R., & McCoy, G. (1991). A preliminary investigation of prediction of mean arterial pressure after self-regulatory treatments. *Biofeedback and Self-Regulation*, 16(2), 181–190.

Blanchard, E. B., Andrasik, F., Neff, D. F., Arena, J. G., Ahles, T. A., Jurish, S. E., et al. (1982). Biofeedback and relaxation training with three kinds of headaches: Treatment effects and their prediction. *Journal of Consulting and Clinical Psychology*, 50(4), 562–575.

Blanchard, E. B., McCoy, G. C., Berger, M., Musso, A., Pallmeyer, T. P., Gerardi, R., et al. (1989). A controlled comparison of thermal biofeedback and relaxation training in the treatment of essential hypertension IV: Prediction of short-term clinical outcome. *Behavior Therapy*, 20(3), 405–415.

Blanchard, E. B., & Schwartz, S. P. (1988). Clinically significant changes in behavior. *Medical Behavior Assessment* (10), 171–188.

Blee, C. (1996). Becoming a racist: Women in contemporary Klu Klux Klan and neo-Nazi groups. *Gender and Society*, 10(6), 680–702.

Bosma, H., Peter, R., Siegrist, J., & Marmot, M. (1998). Two alternative job stress models and the risk of coronary heart disease. *American Journal of Public Health*, 8(2), 68–74.

Botvin, G. J., Schinke, S. P., Epstein, J. A., & Diaz, T. (1994, June). Effectiveness of culturally focused and generic skills training approaches to alcohol and drug abuse prevention among minority youths. *Psychology of Addictive Behaviors*, 8(2), 116–127.

Botvin, G. J., Schinke, S. P., Epstein, J. A., Diaz, T., & Botvin, E. M. (1995, September). Effectiveness of culturally focused and generic skills training approaches to alcohol and drug abuse prevention among minority adolescence: Two-year follow-up results. *Psychology of Addictive Behaviors*, 9(3), 183–194.

Bray, G. A. (1976). The overweight patient. *Advances in Internal Medicine*, 21, 267–308.

Brenner, J. (1973). Factors influencing the specificity of voluntary control. In I. Dicara (Ed.), *Recent advances in limbic and autonomic nervous system research*. New York: Plenum.

Breslau, N., Peterson, E. L., Schultz, L. R., Chilcoat, H. D., & Adreski, P. (1998). Major depression and stages of smoking: A longitudinal investigation. *Archives of General Psychiatry*, 55(1), 161–166.

Brownell, K. D. (1982a, Summer). Exercise and obesity. *Behavioral Medicine Update*, 4(1), 7–11.

Brownell, K. D. (1982b). Behavioral medicine. *Annual Review of Behavior Therapy: Theory and Practice*, 8, 156–207.

Brownell, K. D. (1982c, December). Obesity: Understanding and treating a serious, prevalent, and refractory disorder. *Journal of Consulting and Clinical Psychology*, 50(6), 820–840.

Brownell, K. D., Stunkard, A. J., & Albaum, J. M. (1980). Evaluation and modification of exercise patterns in the natural environment. *American Journal of Psychiatry*, 137, 1540–1545.

Brownell, K. D., & Wadden, T. (1986). Behavior therapy for obesity: Modern approaches and better results. In K. D. Brownell & J. P. Foreyt (Eds.), *Handbook of eating disorders: Physiology, psychology, and treatment of obesity, anorexia and bulimia* (pp. 180–198). New York: Basic Books.

Burns, J. W., Johnson, B. J., Devine, J., Mahoney, N., & Pawl, R. (1998). Anger management style and the prediction of treatment outcomes among male and female chronic pain patients. *Behavior Research and Therapy*, 36, 1051–1062.

Byrne, D. G. (1989a). Personal assessments of life-event stress and the near future onset of psychological symptoms. In T. W. Miller (Ed.), *Stressful life events* (pp. 165–179). Madison, CT: International Universities Press.

Byrne, D. G. (1989b). Personal determinants of life-event stress and myocardial infarction. In T. W. Miller (Ed.), *Stressful life events* (pp. 223–235). Madison, CT: International Universities Press.

Carter, W. B. (1990). Health behavior as a rational process: Theory of reasoned action and multi-attribute utility theory. In K. Glanz, F. M. Lewis, & B. K. Rimer (Eds.), *Health behavior and health education: Theory research and practice* (pp. 63–91). San Francisco, CA: Jossey-Bass Publishers.

Cautela, J. R. (1970). Covert reinforcement. *Behavior Therapy*, 1, 33–50.

Cautela, J. R. (1971). Covert extinction. *Behavior Therapy*, 2, 192–200.

Cautela, J. R. (1973). Covert processes and behavior modification. *Journal of Nervous and Mental Disease*, 157, 27–36.

Chesler, M., & Barbarin, O. (1988). Childhood cancer and the family. *Health and Social Work*, 13(3), 238.

Cinciripini, P. M., & Floreen, A. (1982). An evaluation of a behavioral program for chronic pain. *Journal of Behavioral Medicine*, 5, 375–388.

Cinciripini, P. M., Williamson, D. A., & Epstein, L. H. (1981). The behavioral treatment of migraine headaches. In J. M. Ferguson & C. B. Taylor (Eds.), *The Comprehensive handbook of behavioral medicine* (pp. 207–227). Jamaica, NY: Spectrum Press.

Clark, M. M., Niaura, R., King, T., & Pera, V. (1996). Depression, smoking activity level, and health status: Pretreatment predictors of attrition in obesity treatment. *Addictive Behaviors*, 21(4), 509–513.

Clark, M. M., Pera, V., Goldstein, M. G., Thebarge, R. W., & Guise, B. J. (1996). Counseling strategies for obese patients. *American Journal of Preventive Medicine*, 12(4), 266–270.

Clausen, J. P. (1976, May–June). Circulatory adjustments to dynamic exercise and effect of physical training in normal subjects and in patients with coronary artery disease. *Progress in Cardiovascular Diseases*, 18(6), 459–495.

COMMIT Research Group (1995). Community intervention trial for smoking cessation I. Cohort results from a four-year community intervention. *American Journal of Public Health*, 85(2), 183–192.

Contrada, R. J. (1989, November). Type A behavior, personality hardiness, and cardiovascular responses to stress. *Journal of Personality and Social Psychology*, 57(5), 895–903.

Coulter, M. L., & Hancock, T. (1989). Integrating social work and public health education: A clinical model. *Health and Social Work*, 14(3), 157–164.

Craighead, L. W., & Blum, M. D. (1989). Supervised exercise in behavioral treatment for moderate obesity. *Behavior Therapy*, 20(1), 49–59.

Curry, S. J., Grothaus, L. C., McAfee, T., & Pabiniak, C. (1998). Use and cost-effectiveness of smoking cessation services under four insurance plans in a health maintenance organization. *The New England Journal of Medicine*, 339(10), 673–679.

Curry, S. J., Grothaus, L. C., & McBride, C. (1997). Reasons for quitting: Intrinsic and extrinsic motivations for smoking cessation in a population-based sample of smokers. *Addictive Behaviors*, 22(6), 727–739.

Danielson, R., & Wanzel R. (1977). Exercise objectives of fitness progam droupouts. In D. Landers (Ed.), *Psychology of motor behavior and sport* (pp. 310–320). Champaign, IL: Human Kinetics.

Davidson, R. J., & Schwartz, G. E. (1976a). Matching relaxation therapies to types of anxiety: A patterning approach. In J. White & J. Fadiman (Eds.), *Relax.* New York: Dell Books.

Davidson, R. J., & Schwartz, G. E. (1976b). Relaxation and related states: A bibliography of psychological and physiological research. In J. White & J. Fadiman (Eds.), *Relax.* New York: Dell Books.

Davidson, R. J., & Schwartz, G. E. (1976c). The psychobiology of relaxation and related states: A multi-process theory. In D. I. Mostofsky (Ed.), *Behavior control and the modification of physiological activity* (pp. 399–442). New York: Prentice Hall.

DeAngelis, T. (2005, March). Shaping evidence-based practice. *Monitor on Psychology,* 36(3), 26–31.

Department of Health and Human Services (2003a, May). Frequently asked questions about health problems in African American women. What health problems affect a lot of African American women?

Department of Health and Human Services. (2003b, May). Frequently asked questions about health problems in Asian American/Pacific islander and native Hawaiian women. Who are Asian American/Pacific Islander and native Hawaiian women in the United States? Retrieved November 19, 2008, from http://www.hawaii.edu/ hivandaids/FAQ_about_Health_Problems_in_API_and_Native_Hawaiian_Women. pdf.

Department of Health and Human Services. (2003c, May). Frequently asked questions about health problems in Hispanic American/Latino women. Who are Hispanic American/Latino women in the United States? Retrieved November 19, 2008, from http://www.4women.gov/faq/latina.htm.

Department of Health and Human Services. (2005, January). Frequently asked questions about physical activity (exercise). How can physical activity improve my health?

Dishman, R. K., Oldenburg, B., O'Neal, H., & Shepard, R. J. (1998). Work site physical activity interventions. *Preventive Medicine,* 15(4), 344–361.

Drougas, H. J., Reed, G., & Hill, J. O. (1992). Comparison of dietary self-reports with energy expenditure measured using a whole room indirect calorimeter. *Journal of the American Dietetic Association,* 92, 1073–1077.

Durbeck, D. C., Heinzelmann, F., Schacter, J., Haskell, W. L., Payne, G. H., Moxley, R. T., III, et al. (1972, November). The national aeronautics and space administration—U.S. public health service health evaluation and enhancement program. Summary of results. *The American Journal of Cardiology,* 30(7), 784–790.

Edmunds, M. (1998). Health care policy. In E. Blechman & K. Brownell (Eds.), *Behavioral medicine for women: A comprehensive handbook.* New York: Guilford Publications.

Eisenberg, D. M., Delbanco, T. L, Berkey, C. S, Kaptuchuk, T. J., Kupelnick, B., Kuhl, J., et al. (1993). Cognitive behavioral techniques for hypertension: Are they effective? *Annals of Internal Medicine,* 118(12), 964–972.

Eiser, J. R., & Sutton, S. R. (1979). Smoking, seat-belts, and beliefs about health. *Addictive Behaviors,* 4(4), 331–338.

El-Askari, G., Freestone, J., Irizarry C., Draut, K. L., Mashiyama, S. T., Morgan, M. A., et al. (1998). The healthy neighborhoods project: A local health departments role in catalyzing community development. *Health Education and Behavior,* 25(2), 146–159.

Eliahou, H. E., Iaina, A., Gaon, T., Shochat, J., & Modan, M. (1981). Body weight reduction necessary to attain normotension in the overweight hypertensive patient. *International Journal of Obesity*, 5(Suppl. 1), 157–163.

Elixhauser, A. (1990). The costs of smoking and the cost-effectiveness of smoking cessation programs. *Journal of Public Health Policy*, 11(2), 218–237.

Fahrion, S., Norris, P., Green, A., Green, E., & Snarr, C. (1986). Biobehavioral treatment of essential hypertension: A group outcome study. *Biofeedback and Self-Regulation*, 11(4), 257–279.

Fernandez, E., & Sheffield, J. (1996). Relative contributions of life events versus daily hassles to the frequency and intensity of headaches. *Headache*, 36, 595–602.

Field, A. E., Coakley, E. H., Must, A., Spadano, J. L., Laird, N., Dietz, W. H., et al. (2001). Impact of overweight on the risk of developing common chronic diseases during a 10-year period. *Archives of Internal Medicine*, 161(13), 1581–1586.

Fishbein, M. (1967). Attitude and the prediction of behavior: Results of a survey sample. In M. Fishbein (Ed.), *Readings in attitude theory and measurement*. New York: Wiley.

Fletcher, G. F., Balady, G., Froelicher, V. F., Hartley, L. H., Haskell, W. L., & Pollock, M. L. (1995). Exercise standards: A statement for health care professionals from the American Heart Association. *Circulation*, 91(2), 596–601.

Folkins, C. H., & Sime, W. E. (1981). Physical fitness training and mental health. *American Psychologist*, 36(4), 373–389.

Forester, J. L., Murray, D. M., Wolfson, M., Blaine, T. M., Wagenaar, A. C., & Hennrikus, D. J. (1998). The effects of community policies to reduce youth access to tobacco. *American Journal of Public Health*, 88(8), 1193–1198.

Foreyt, J. P., Ramirez, A. G., & Cousins, J. H. (1991). Cuidando El Corazon— a weight-reduction intervention for Mexican Americans. *American Journal of Clinical Nutrition*, 53, 1639S–1641S.

Forgey, M. A., Schinke, S., & Cole, K. (1997). School-based interventions to prevent substance use among inner-city minority adolescents. In D. K. Wilson, J. R. Rodriguez, & W. C. Taylor (Eds.), *Health-promoting and health-compromising behaviors among minority adolescents. Applications and practice in health psychology* (pp. 251–267). Washington, DC: American Psychological Association.

Frederiksen, L. W., & Simon, S. J. (1978a). Modification of smoking topography: A preliminary analysis. *Behavioral Therapy*, 9, 946–949.

Frederiksen, L. W., & Simon, S. J. (1978b, Fall). Modifying how people smoke: Instructional control and generalization. *Journal of Applied Behavior Analysis*, 11(3), 431–432.

French, D. J., Gauthier J. G., Roberge, C., Bouchard, S., & Nouwen, A. (1997). Self-efficacy in the thermal biofeedback treatment of migraine sufferers. *Behavior Therapy*, 28(1), 109–125.

Furguson, R. J., & Ahles, T. A. (1998). Private body consciousness, anxiety and pain symptoms reports of chronic pain and patients. *Behavior Research and Therapy*, 36, 527–535.

Gagliese, L., & Melzack, R. (1997). Chronic pain in elderly people. *Pain*, 70, 3–14.

Ganley, R. M. (1988). Emotional eating and how it relates to dietary restraint, disinhibition and perceived hunger. *International Journal of Eating Disorders*, 7, 635–647.

Glantz, K., Lewis, F. M., & Rimer, B. K. (1990). *Health behavior and health education: Theory research and practice* (p. 25). San Francisco, CA: Jossey-Bass Publishers.

Glasgow, M. S., Engel, B. T., & D'Lugoff, B. C. (1989). A controlled study of a standardized behavioral stepped treatment for hypertension. *Psychosomatic Medicine,* 51(1), 10–26.

Glasgow, M. S., Gaardner, K. R., & Engel, B. T. (1982). Behavioral treatment of high blood Pressure. II. Acute and sustained effects of relaxation and systolic blood pressure biofeedback. *Psychosomatic Medicine,* 44, 155–170.

Goldman, L. K., & Glantz, S. A. (1998). Evaluation of anti-smoking advertising. *Journal of the American Medical Association,* 279 (10), 772–777.

Haas, A. L., Munoz, R. F., Humfleet, G. L., Reus, V. I., & Hall, S. M. (2004). Influences of mood, depression history, and treatment modality on outcomes in smoking cessation. *Journal of Consulting and Clinical Psychology,* 72(4), 563–570. Retrieved on February, 26, 2005, from http://contentapa.org/journals/ccp/72/4/563.html.

Hall, S. M., Munoz, R. F., & Reus, V. I. (1994). Cognitive-behavioral intervention increases abstinence rates for depressive-history smokers. *Journal of Consulting and Clinical Psychology,* 62, 141–146.

Harlow, S. D., Bainbridge, K., Howard, D., Myntti, C., Potter, L., Sussman, N., et al. (1999). Methods and measures: Emerging strategies in women's health research. *Journal of Women's Health,* 8(2), 139–144.

Heirich, M. A., Foote, A., Erfurt, J. C., & Konopka, B. (1993, May). Worksite physical fitness programs. Comparing the impact of different program designs on cardiovascular risks. *Journal of Occupational Medicine,* 35(5), 510–517.

Heitmann, B. L. (1993, June). The influence of fatness, weight change, slimming history and other lifestyle variables on diet reporting in Danish men and women aged 35–65 years. *International Journal of Obesity Related Metabolic Disorders,* 17(6), 329–336.

Helstrom, A. W., Coffey, C., & Jorgannathan, P. (1998). Asian-American women's health. In E. Blechman & K. Brownell (Eds.), *Behavioral medicine for women: A comprehensive handbook.* (pp. 826–832). New York: Guilford Publications.

Hochbaum, G. (1958). *Public participation in medical screening programs: A sociopsychological study.* U.S. Public Health Service Publication No. 572. Washington, DC: U.S. Government Printing Office.

Hollis, J. F., Lichtenstein, E., Vogt, T. M., Stevens, V. J., & Biglan, A. (1993). Nurse assisted counseling for smokers in primary care. *Annals of Internal Medicine,* 118, 521–525

Holm, J. E., Bury, L., & Suda, K. T. (1996). The relationship between stress, headache, and the menstrual cycle in young female migraineurs. *Headache,* 36(9), 531–537.

Holroyd, K. A., & Andrasik, F. (1982). A cognitive-behavioral approach to recurrent tension and migraine headache. In P. Kendall (Ed.), *Advances in cognitive-behavioral research and therapy* (pp. 276–320). New York: Academic Press.

Horton, E. W. (1981). The role of exercise in the treatment of hypertension in obesity. *International Journal of Obesity,* 5 (Suppl.), 165–171.

Hudmon, K. S., Gritz, E. R., Clayton, S., & Nisenbaum, R. (1999). Eating orientation, postcessation weight gain, and continued abstinence among female smokers receiving an unsolicited smoking cessation intervention. *Health Psychology,* 18(1), 29–36. Retrieved February 26, 2005, from http://content.apa.org/journals/hea/18/1/29.html.

Hughes, J. R. (1996). The future of smoking cessation therapy in the United States. *Addiction*, 91(12), 1797–1802.

Ivancevich, J. M. (1986). Life events and hassles as predictors of health symptoms, job performance and absenteeism. *Journal of Occupational Behavior Therapy*, 7, 39–51.

Jason, L. A., & McMahon, S. D. (1998). Stress and coping in smoking cessation: A longitudinal examination. *Academic Search Premier*, 11. Retrieved April 1, 2005, from http://web23.epnetcom.proxy.lib.utk.edu:90/citation.asp?tb=1&_ug=sid+9519.

Jackson, Y., Dietz, W. H., Sanders, C., Kolbe, L. J., Whyte, J. J., Wechsler, H., et al. (2002). Summary of the 2000 Surgeon General's listening session: Toward a national action plan on overweight and obesity. *Obesity Research*, 10, 1299–1305. Retrieved April, 10, 2005, from http://www.obesityresearch.org/cgi/content/full/10/12/1299.

Janz, N. K., & Becker, M. H. (1984). The health belief model: A decade later. *Health Education Quarterly*, 11, 1–47.

Jeffery, R. W., & French, S. A. (1997). Preventing weight gain in adults: Design, methods and one year results from the pound of prevention study. *International Journal of Obesity and Related Metabolic Disorders*, 21(6), 457–464.

Jeffery, R. W., Vender, M., & Wing, R. R. (1978). Weight loss and behavior change 1 year after behavioral treatment for obesity. *Journal of Consulting and Clinical Psychology*, 46(2), 368–369.

Jenkins, C. N., McPhee, S. J., Bird, J. A., Pham, G. Q., Nguyen, B. H., Lai, K. Q., et al. (1999). Effect of a media-led education campaign on breast and cervical cancer screening among Vietnamese-American women. *Preventative Medicine*, 28(4), 395–406.

Johnsen, L., Spring, B., Pingitore, R., Sommerfeld, B. K., & MacKirnan, D. (2002). Smoking as subculture? Influence on Hispanic and non-Hispanic white women's attitudes toward smoking and obesity. *Health Psychology*, 21(3), 279–287. Retrieved February 26, 2005, from http://content.apa.org.proxy.lib.utk.edu:90/journals/hea/21/3/279.html.

Kannel, W. B., & Sorlie, P. (1979, August). Some health benefits of physical activity. The Framingham Study. *Archives of Internal Medicine*, 139(8), 857–861.

Kaplan, R. M., Sallis, J. E., & Patterson, T. I. (1993). *Health and human behavior*, pp. 39–86. New York: McGraw-Hill.

Keefe, F. J. (1982, December). Behavioral assessment and treatment of chronic pain: Current status and future directions. *Journal of Consulting and Clinical Psychology*, 50(6), 896–911.

Keefe, F. J., Brown, C., Scott, D. S., & Ziesat, H. (1982). Behavioral assessment of chronic pain. In F. J. Keefe & J. A. Blumenthal (Eds.), *Assessment strategies in behavioral medicine* (pp. 321–350). New York: Grune & Stratton.

Keefe, F. J., Dunsmore, L., & Burnett, R. (1992). Behavioral and cognitive behavioral approaches to chronic pain: Recent advances and future directions. *Journal of Consulting and Clinical Psychology*, 60, 528–536.

Kendrick, J. S., & Merritt, R. K. (1996). Women and smoking: An update for the 1990s. *American Journal of Obstetrics and Gynecology*, 175(3), 528–535.

Keys, A. (1980, September). W. O. Atwater memorial lecture: Overweight, obesity, coronary heart disease and mortality. *Nutrition Reviews*, 38(9), 297–307.

Kowal, N. R. (2001). Beyond invasive therapy: Chronic nonmalignant pain and the cognitive-behavioral perspective. *AAACN Viewpoint.* Retrieved November 19, 2008, from http://findarticles.com/p/articles/mi_qa4022/is_200109?pnum=4&opg=n8959324&tag=artBody;col1.

Kristiansen, C. M. (1985). Smoking, health behavior, and value priorities. *Addictive Behaviors, 10*(1), 41–44.

Kuczmarski, R. J., & Flegal, K. M. (1994). Increasing prevalence of overweight among U.S. adults. *Journal of the American Medical Association, 272*(3), 205–211.

Kumanyika, S. (1995). Nutrition & health campaign for all women. *Journal of the American Dietetic Association, 95*(3), 299–300.

Labbe, E., Murphy, E., & O'Brien, L. (1996). Psychological factors and prediction of headaches in college adults. *Headache, 37,* 1–5.

Lando, H. A. (1981). Effects of preparation, experimenter contact, and a maintained reduction alternative on a broad-spectrum program for eliminating smoking. *Addictive Behaviors, 6,* 123–133.

Lando, H. A., & McGovern, P. G. (1982). Three-year data on a behavioral treatment for smoking: A follow-up note. *Addictive Behaviors, 7*(2), 177–181.

Lang, P. (1974). Learned control of heart rate in a computer directed environment. In P. Obrist, A. Black, J. Brener, & L. DiCara, (Eds), *Contemporary trends in cardiovascular psychophysiology* (pp. 392–405). Chicago, IL: Aldine-Atherton.

Leon, A. S., & Blackburn, H. (1977). The relationship of physical activity to coronary heart disease and life expectancy. *Annals of the New York Academy of Sciences, 301,* 561–578.

Lehrer, P. M., Carr, R., Sargunaraj, D., & Woolfold, R. L. (1994). Stress management techniques: Are they all equivalent, or do they have specific effects? *Biofeedback and Self-Regulation, 19*(4), 353–401.

Leukefeld, C. G. (1989). The future of social work in public health. *Health and Social Work, 14*(1), 9–11.

Levenstein, S., Smith, M. W., & Kaplan, G. A. (2001). Psychosocial predictors of hypertension in men and women. *Archives of Internal Medicine, 161,* 1341–1346. Retrieved February 26, 2005, from http://americanmedicalassociation.com.

Levy, B. T., & Williamson, P. S. (1988). Patient perceptions and weight loss of obese adults. *Journal of Family Practice, 27*(3), 285–290.

Lewis, C. E., Smith, D. E., Wallace, D. D., Williams, O. D., Bild, D. E., & Jacobs, D. R. (1997). Seven-year trends in body weight and associations with lifestyle and behavioral characteristics in black and white young adults: The CARDIA study. *American Journal of Public Health, 87*(40), 635–642.

Lichtenstein, E. (1982). The smoking problem: A behavioral perspective. *Journal of Consulting and Clinical Psychology, 50*(6), 804–819.

Lichtenstein, E., Biglan, A., Glasgow, R. E., Severson, H., & Ary, D. (1990). The tobacco use research program at Oregon Research Institute. *British Journal of Addictions, 85,* 715–724.

Lichtenstein, E., Hollis, J. F., Severson, H. H., Stevens, V. J., Vogt, T. M., Glasgow, R. E., et al. (1996). Tobacco cessation interventions in health care settings: Rationale, model, outcomes. *Addictive Behaviors, 21*(6), 709–720.

Lichtenstein, E., & Mermelstein, R. J. (1986). Some methodological cautions in the use of the tolerance questionnaire. *Addictive Behaviors, 11*(4), 439–442.

Lichtman, S. W., Pisarska, K., Berman, E. R., Prestone, M., Dowling, H., Offenbacher, E., et al. (1992). Discrepancy between self-reported and actual food intake and exercise in obese subjects. *New England Journal of Medicine, 327,* 1893–1898.

Linden, W., & Chambers L. (1994). Clinical effectiveness of non-drug treatment for hypertension: A meta-analysis. *Annals of Behavioral Medicine*, 16, 35–45.

Livingstone, M. B. E., Pretice, A. M., Coward, W. A., Strain, J. J., Black, A. E., Barker, M. E., et al. (1990). Accuracy of weighed dietary records in studies of diet and health. *British Medical Journal*, 300, 708–712.

MacKenzie, T. D., Bartecchi, C. E., & Schrier, R. W. (1994). The human cost of tobacco use. *New England Journal of Medicine*, 330, 975–980.

Maffeis, C., Shultz, Y., Zafanello, M., Piccoli, R., & Pinelli, L. (1994). Elevated energy expenditure and reduced energy intake in obese prepubertal children: Paradox of poor dietary reliability in obesity. *Journal of Pediatrics*, 124, 348–345.

Mahoney, E. R. (1974a). Body-cathexis and self-esteem: The importance of subjective importance. *Journal of Psychology: Interdisciplinary and Applied*, 88(1), 27–30.

Mahoney, K. (1974b). Count on it: A simple self-monitoring device. *Behavior Therapy*, 5(5), 701–703.

Mahoney, M. J. (1974c). Self-reward and self-monitoring techniques for weight control. *Behavior Therapy*, 5(1), 48–57.

Mahoney, M. J. (1974d). *Cognition and behavior modification*. Oxford, England: Ballinger.

Makail, S. F., & von Baeyer, C. L. (1990). Pain, somatic focus and emotional adjustment in children of chronic headache sufferers and controls. *Social Science and Medicine*, 31, 51–59.

Mann, G. V., Garrett, H. L., Farhi, A., Murray H., & Billings, F. T. (1969). Exercise to prevent coronary heart disease. An experimental study of the effects of training on risk factors for coronary disease in men. *The American Journal of Medicine*, 46(1), 12–27.

Marcus B. H., Emmons, K. M., Simkin-Silverman, L. R., Linnan, L. A., Taylor, E. R., Bock, B. C., et al. (1998). Evaluation of motivationally tailored vs. standard self-help physical activity interventions at the workplace. *American Journal of Health Promotion*, 12(4), 246–253.

Marshack, E., Davidson K., & Mizrahi, T. (1988, Summer). Preparation of social workers for a changing health care environment. *Health and Social Work*, 13(3), 226–233.

Martin, J. E., & Dubbert, P. M. (1982). Exercise applications and promotion in behavioral medicine: Current status and future directions. *Journal of Consulting and Clinical Psychology*, 50(6), 1004–1017.

Martin, P. R., & Theunissen, C. (1993). The role of life event stress, coping and social support in chronic headaches. *Headache*, 33, 301–306.

Martinson, B. C., O'Conner, P. J., & Pronk, N. P. (2001). Physical inactivity and short-term all-cause mortality in adults with chronic disease. *Archives of Internal Medicine*, 161, 1173–1180.

McClelland, D. C. (1989). Motivational factors in health and disease. *American Psychologist*, 44(40), 675–683.

McGrady, A., & Roberts, G. (1992). Racial differences in the relaxation response of hypertensives. *Psychosomatic Medicine*, 54(1), 71–78.

McNair, L. D., & Roberts, G. W. (1998). African-American women's health. In E. A. Blechman & K. D. Brownell (Eds.), *Behavioral medicine and women: A comprehensive handbook* (pp. 821–825). New York: Guilford Publications.

McRae, B. C., & Choi-Lao, A. (1978). National survey on smoking and health education in prenatal classes in Canada. *Canadian Journal of Public Health*, 69(6), 427–430.

Moncher, M. S., Holden, G. W., & Schinke, S. S. (1991, April). Psychosocial correlates of adolescent substance use: A review of current etiological constructs.
International Journal of the Addictions, 26(4), 377–414.

Mongini, F., Defilippi, N., & Negro, C. (1996). Chronic daily headache: A clinical
and psychosocial profile before and after treatment. *Headache*, 37, 83–87.

Montano, D. E., Kasprzyk, D., & Taplin, S. H. (1997). The theory of reasoned action
and the theory of planned behavior. In K. Glanz, F. M. Lewis, & B. K. Rimer (Eds.),
Health behavior and health education: Theory, research, and practice (2nd ed.,
pp. 85–113). San Francisco, CA: Jossey-Bass Publishers.

NIH Technology Assessment Panel (1996). Integration of behavioral and relaxation
approaches into the treatment of chronic pain and insomnia. *Journal of the American
Medical Association*, 276(4), 313–318.

Niaura, R., & Abrams, D. B. (2002). Smoking cessation progress, priorities, and
prospectus. *Journal of Consulting and Clinical Psychology*, 70(3), 494–509. Retrieved
February 26, 2005, from http://contentapa.org/journals/ccp/70/3/494.html.

Ockene, J. K., & Zapka, J. G. (1997). Physician-based smoking intervention: A re-
dedication to a five-step strategy to smoking research. *Addictive Behaviors*, 22(6),
835–848.

Orme-Johnson, D. (1987). Medical care utilization and the transcendental meditation
program. *Psychosomatic Medicine*, 49, 493–507.

Packard, E. (2005, December). From basic research to health-care messages: Improved
public health is a priority for many APA Div. 8 social psychologists. *Monitor on
Psychology*, 84–85.

Paine-Andrews, A., Harris, K. J., Fawcett, S. B., Richter, K. P., Lewis, R. K., Francisco,
V. T., et al. (1997). Evaluating a statewide partnership for reducing risks for chronic
disease. *Journal of Community Health*, 22(5), 373–379.

Pallonen, U. E., Velicer, W. F., Prochaska, J. O., Rossi, F. S., Bellis, J. M., Tsoh,
J. Y., et al. (1998). Computer-based smoking cessation interventions in adolescents:
Description, feasibility, and six-month follow-up findings. *Substance Use & Misuse*,
33(4), 935–965.

Patel, C., & North, W. R. (1975). Randomized control trial of yoga and biofeedback
in the management of hypertension. *Lancet*, 2(1), 93–95.

Pekkarinen, T., & Mustajoki, P. (1997). Comparison of behavior therapy with and
without very-low-energy diet in the treatment of morbid obesity: A 5-year outcome.
Archives of Internal Medicine, 157(14), 1581–1585.

Perttula, W., Lowe, D., & Quon, N. S. (1999). Asian American health care attitudes.
Health Marketing Quarterly, 16(2), 39–53.

Peterson, T. R., & Aldana, S. G. (1999). Improving exercise behavior: An application
of the stages of change model in a worksite setting. *American Journal of Health
Promotion*, 13(4), 229–232.

Pickering, J. E. (1982, September). Nutritional and pharmacologic management of
hyperlipoproteinemia. *Angiology*, 33(9), 577–580.

Pinkerton, S., Hughes, N., & Wenrich, W. (1982). *Behavioral medicine: Clinical
applications*. New York: Wiley.

Pomerleau, O. F. (1981). Underlying mechanisms in substance abuse: Examples from
research on smoking. *Addictive Behaviors*, 6, 187–196.

Prochaska, J. O. (1996). A stage paradigm for integrating clinical and public health
approaches to smoking cessation. *Addictive Behaviors*, 21(60), 721–732.

Prochaska, J. O., & DeClemente, C. G. (1983). Stages and processes of self-change of smoking: Toward an integrative model of change. *Journal of Consulting and Clinical Psychology*, 51, 390–395.

Prochaska, J. O., Norcross, J. C., & DeClemente, C. G. (1994). *Changing for good: A revolutionary six stage program for overcoming bad habits and moving your life positively forward.* New York: Avon Books.

Prochaska, J. O., Redding, C. A., & Evers, K. E. (1997). The trans-theoretical model and stages of change. In K. Glanz, F. M. Lewis, & B. K. Rimer (Eds.), *Health behavior and health education: Theory, research and practice* (2nd ed., pp. 60–84). San Fransisco, CA: Jossey-Bass Publishers.

Rabois, D., & Haaga, D. A. F. (1997a). Cognitive coping, history of depression, and cigarette smoking. *Addictive Behaviors*, 22(6), 789–796.

Rabois, D., & Haaga, D. A. F. (1997b). Cognitive coping, history of depression, and brief smoking cessation program following reinforcement contact after training: A randomized trial. *Preventative Medicine*, 27, 77–83.

Raines, J. W., & Erickson, G. (1997). Putting prevention into practice. *Journal of Professional Nursing*, 13(2), 124–128.

Richmond, R., Mendelsohn, C., & Kehoe, L. (1998). Family physicians' utilization of a brief smoking cessation program following reinforcement contact after training: A randomized trial. *Preventative Medicine*, 27, 77–83.

Rigotti, N. A. (1999). Treatment options for the weight-conscious smoker. *Archives of Internal Medicine*, 159, 1169–1171. Retrieved on February 26, 2005, from http://americanmedical association.com.

Rigotti, N. A., Arnsten, J. H., McKool, K. M., Wood-Reid, K. M., Pasternak, R. C., & Singer, D. E. (1997). Efficacy of a smoking cessation program for hospital patients. *Archive of Internal Medicine*, 8(22), 2653–2660.

Roberts, G., & McGrady, A. (1996). Racial and gender effects on the relaxation response: Implications for the development of hypertension. *Biofeedback and Self-Regulation*, 21(1), 51–62.

Rosenstock, I. M. (1990). The health belief model: Explaining health behavior through expectancies. In K. Glanz, L. Marcus, & B. Rimer (Eds.), *Health behavior and health education: Theory research and practice* (pp. 39–62). San Francisco, CA: Jossey-Bass.

Rosenstock, I. M., & Kirscht, J. P. (1974). The health belief model and personal health behavior. *Health Education Monographs*, 2, 470–473.

Roskies, E. (1987). *Stress management for the healthy type A. A skills training program.* New York: Guilford Press.

Roth, D. L., & Holmes, D. S. (1987). Influence of aerobic exercise training and relaxation training on physical and psychological health following stressful life events. *Psychosomatic Medicine*, 49, 355–365.

Ruiter, R. A. C., Kessels, L. T. E., Jansma, B. M., & Brug, J. (2006). Increased attention for computer-tailored health communications: An event-related potential study. *Health Psychology*, 25(3), 300–306.

Sallis, J. F. (1998). Reflections on the physical activity intervention conference. *American Journal of Preventative Medicine*, 15(4), 431–432.

Sallis, J. F., Bauman, A., & Pratt, M. (1998). Environmental and policy interventions to promote physical activity. *American Journal of Preventive Medicine*, 15(4), 379–397.

Sanders, S. H. (1979, April). A trimodal behavioral conceptualization of clinical pain. *Perceptual and Motor Skills*, 48(2), 551–555.

Schachter, S. (1977). Nicotine regulation in heavy and light smokers. *Journal of Experimental Psychology: General*, 106, 5–12.

Scheurer, J., & Tipton, C. M. (1977). Cardiovascular adaptations to physical training. *Annual Review of Physiology*, 39, 221–251.

Schoeller, D. A. (1990). How accurate is self-reported dietary energy intake? *Nutrition Review*, 48, 373–387.

Schwartz, G. E., Weinberger D. A., & Singer, J. A. (1981). Cardiovascular differentiation of happiness, sadness, anger, and fear following imagery and exercise. *Psychosomatic Medicine*, 43(4), 343–364.

Shannon, P. (1989). Basal readers: Three perspectives. *Theory into Practice*, 28(4), 235–239.

Shapiro, D., & Goldstein, I. B. (1982). Biobehavioral perspectives on hypertension. *Journal of Consulting and Clinical Psychology*, 50(6), 841–858.

Shepard, A. J. (1997). Exercise and relaxation health promotion. *Sports Medicine*, 23(40), 211–217.

Silver, B. V., & Blanchard, E. B. (1978). Biofeedback and relaxation training in the treatment of psychophysiological disorders: Or are the machines really necessary. *Journal of Behavioral Medicine*, 1(2), 217–239.

Smith, J. C., Amutio, A., Anderson, J. P., & Aria, L. A. (1996). Relaxation: Mapping an uncharted world. *Biofeedback and Self Regulation*, 21(1), 63–90.

Soman, V. R., Koivisto, V. A., Deibert, D., Felig, P., & DeFronzo, R. A. (1979). Increased insulin sensitivity and insulin binding to monocytes after physical training. *The New England Journal of Medicine*, 301(22), 1200–1204.

Sorensen, G., Lewis, B., & Bishop, R. (1996). Gender, job factors, and coronary heart disease risk. *American Journal of Health Behavior*, 21(1), 3–13.

Speers, M. A., & Lancaster, B. (1998). Disease prevention and health promotion in urban areas: CDC's perspective. *Health Education and Behavior*, 25(2), 226–233.

Stalonas, P. M., Johnson, W. G., & Christ, M. (1978, June). Behavior modification for obesity: The evaluation of exercise, contingency management, and program adherence. *Journal of Consulting and Clinical Psychology*, 46(3), 463–469.

Stalonas, P. M., Perri, M. G., & Kerzner, A. B. (1984). Do behavioral treatments of obesity last? A five-year follow-up investigation. *Addictive Behavior*, 9(2), 175–183.

Stamler, J. F., Brody, M. J., & Phillips, M. I. (1980, March). The central and peripheral effects of Captopril (SQ 14225) on the arterial pressure of the spontaneously hypertensive rat. *Brain Research*, 186(2), 499–503.

Stevens, V. J., Glasgow, E., Hollis, J. F., Lichtenstein, E., & Vogt, T. M. (1993). A smoking-cessation intervention for hospital patients. *Medical Care*, 31, 65–72.

Stitzer, M. L., & Bigelow, G. E. (1985). Contingent reinforcement for reduced breath carbon monoxide levels: target-specific effects on cigarette smoking. *Addictive Behaviors*, 10(4), 345–349.

Storer, J. H., Cychosz, C. M., & Anderson, D. F. (1997). Wellness behaviors, social identities, and health promotion. *American Journal of Health Behavior*, 21(4), 260–268.

Subramanian, K., & Rose, S. D. (1988). Social work and the treatment of chronic pain. *Health & Social Work*, 13(1), 49–60.

Taylor, H. L., Buskirk, E. R., & Remingon, R. D. (1973). Exercise in controlled trials of the prevention of coronary heart disease. *Federation Proceedings*, 32(5), 1623–1627.

Taylor, C. B., Coffey, T., Berra, K., Iaffaldano, R., Casey, K., & Haskell, W. L. (1984). Seven-day activity and self-report compared to a direct measure of physical activity. *American Journal of Epidemiology*, 120(6), 818–824.

Todd, M. (2004). Daily processes in stress and smoking effects of negative events, nicotine dependence, and gender. *Psychology of Addictive Behaviors*, 18(1), 31–39. Retrieved February 26, 2005, from http://content.apa.org/journals/adb/18/1/31.html.

U.S. Department of Health and Human Services (USDHHS) (1990). *The health benefits of smoking cessation* (DHHS Publication (DCD) 90–8416). Atlanta, GA: US Department of Health and Human Services, Public Health Services, Centers for Disease Control, Center for Chronic Disease Prevention and Health Promotion, Office on Smoking and Health.

U.S. Department of Health and Human Services (USDHHS) (1991). *Health people 2000* (full report with commentary). Washington, DC: U.S. Government Printing Office; DHHS publication no. (PHS) 91–50212.

U.S. Department of Health and Human Services (USDHHS) (1994). *Preventing tobacco use among young people: A report of the Surgeon General.* Washington, DC: U.S. Department of Health and Human Services, Public Health Service, Center for Disease Control and Prevention, National Center for Chronic Disease Prevention and Health Promotion, Office on Smoking and Health.

U.S. Department of Health, Education, and Welfare (USDHEW) (1979). *Smoking and health: A report of the Surgeon General.* Washington, DC: U.S. Department of Health, Education, and Welfare, Public Health Service, Office of the Assistant Secretary for Health. Office on Smoking and Health, DHEW Publication Number (PHS) 79–50066, pp. 1136.

U.S. Public Health Service (1996). Office of the Surgeon General. *Physical activity and health: A report of the Surgeon General.* Atlanta, GA: U.S. Dept. of Health and Human Services, Centers for Disease Control and Prevention, National Center for Chronic Disease Prevention and Health Promotion.

Van Itallie, T. B. (1986, January). Bad news and good news about obesity. *New England Journal of Medicine*, 314(4), 239–240.

Walcott-McQuigg, J. A. (1995). The relationship between stress and weight-control behavior in African-American women. *Journal of the National Medical Association*, 87(6), 427–432.

Watson, D. L., & Tharp, R. G. (1993). *Self-directed behavior: Self-motivation for personal adjustment* (6th ed.). Pacific Grove, CA: Brooks/Cole Publishing.

Weaver, M., & McGrady, A. (1995). Blood pressure response to biofeedback-assisted relaxation: Can it be predicted? *Biofeedback and Self-Regulation*, 20, 229–240.

Weiner, H. (1979). *Psychobiology of essential hypertension.* New York: Elsevier.

Wetter, D. W., Fiore, M. C., Gritz, E. R., Lando, H. A., Stitzer, M. L., Hasselblad, V., et al. (1998). The Agency for Health Care Policy and Research, smoking cessation clinical guideline: Findings and implications for psychologists. *American Psychologist*, 53(6), 657–699.

Whitlock, E. P., Vogt, T. M., Hollis, J. F., & Lichtenstein, E. (1997). Does gender affect response to a brief clinic-based smoking intervention? *American Journal of Preventive Medicine*, 13(3), 159–166.

Wild, R. A., Taylor, E. L., & Knehans, A. (1995, January). The gynecologist and the prevention of cardiovascular disease. *American Journal of Obstetrics and Gynecology*, 172(1 Pt. 1), 1–13.

Wilhelmsen, L., Sanne, H., Elmfeldt, D., Grimby, G., Tibblin, G., & Wedel, H. (1975). A controlled trial of physical training after myocardial infarction. Effects on risk factors, nonfatal reinfarction, and death. *Preventive Medicine*, 4(4), 491–508.

Williams, S. G., Hudson, A., & Redd, C. (1982). Cigarette smoking, manifest anxiety and somatic symptoms. *Addictive Behaviors*, 7(4), 427–428.

Williamson, D. F. (1995). Prevalence and demographics of obesity. In K. D. Brownell & C. G. Fairburn (Eds.), *Eating disorders and obesity* (pp. 391–395). New York: Guilford Publications.

Wilson, G. T., Franks, C. M., Kendall, P. C., & Foreyt, J. P. (1987). Behavioral medicine: Review of behavioral therapy. *Theory and Practice*, 11, 155–186.

Winerman, L. (2005, November). Exercise may protect against brain-cell loss. *Monitor on Psychology*, 21.

Wodarski, J. S. (1985). *Introduction to human behavior*. Austin, TX: PRO-ED.

Wodarski, J. S. (1989). *Preventive health services for adolescents*. Springfield, IL: Charles C. Thomas.

Wodarski, J. S. (2000). The role for social workers in the managed health care system: Model for empirically based psychosocial interventions. *Crisis Intervention and Time Limited Treatment*, 6(2), 109–140.

Wodarski, J. S., & Bagarozzi, D. A. (1979). *Behavioral social work*. New York: Human Sciences Press.

Wodarski, J. S., & Wodarski, L. A. (1993). *Curriculums and practical aspects of implementation: Preventive health services for adolescents*. Lanham, MD: University Press of America.

Wodarski, J. S., Wodarski, L. A., & Dulmus, C. N. (2003). *Adolescent depression and suicide: A comprehensive empirical intervention for prevention and treatment*. Springfield, IL: Charles C. Thomas.

Wodarski, J. S., Wodarski, L. A., Nixon, S. C., & Mackie, C. M. (1991). Behavioral medicine: An emerging field of social work practice. *Journal of Health and Social Policy*, 3(1), 19–43.

Woodward, A. M. (1998). Hispanic women and health care. In E. Blechman & K. Brownell (Eds.), *Behavioral medicine & women: A comprehensive handbook*. New York: Guilford Press.

Worden, J. K., Flynn, B. S., Solomon, L. J., Secker-Walker, R. H., Badger, G. J., & Carpenter, J. H. (1996). Using mass media to prevent cigarette smoking among adolescent girls. *Health Education Quarterly*, 23(4), 453.

Yates A. J., & Thain J. (1985). Self-efficacy as a predictor of relapse following voluntary cessation of smoking. *Addictive Behaviors*, 10(3), 291–298.

Zamarra, J. W., Schneider, R. H., Besseghini, I., Robinson, D. K., & Salerno, J. W. (1996). Usefulness of the transcendental meditation program in the treatment of patients with coronary artery disease. *The American Journal of Cardiology*, 77, 867–870.

Zarski, J. J. (1994). Hassles and health: A replication. *Health Psychology*, 3, 243–251.

Ziegler, D. K., Hassanein, R. S., & Couch, J. R. (1977). Characteristics of life headache histories in a nonclinic population. *Neurology*, 27(3), 265–269.

Zittel, K. (1999). *Smoking cessation in teenagers: Paradigms and implications for social work practice*. Unpublished manuscript, School of Social Work, State University of New York at Buffalo.

8   Prevention: Cost Saving for Reducing Health Care Costs

Allman, R., Taylor, H. A., & Nathan, P. E. (1972). Group drinking during stress: Effects on drinking behavior. *American Journal of Psychiatry*, 129(6), 45–54.

American Psychology Association (APA) (2006, June). In the public interest: The national push for workplace health. *Monitor on Psychology*, 37(6), 32.

Azrin, N. H. (1978). A learning approach to job finding. Paper presented at the Association for Advancement of Behavior Therapy, Chicago, IL., November 1978.

Bernstein, D. A., & Borkovec, T. D. (1973). *Progressive relaxation training: A manual for the helping professions*. Champaign, IL: Research Press.

Botvin, G. J. (2004). Advancing prevention science and practice: Challenges, critical issues, and future directions. *Prevention Science*, 5(1), 69–72.

Bruce, M. L., Takeuchi, D. T., & Leaf, P. J. (1991). Poverty and psychiatric status: Longitudinal evidence from the New Haven Epidemiologic Catchment Area Study. *Archives of General Psychiatry*, 48, 470–474.

Buxbaum, C. B. (1981). Cost benefit analysis: The mystique versus the reality. *Social Service Review*, 55(3), 453–471.

Caplan, G. (1964). *Principles of preventive psychiatry*. New York: Basic Books.

Castro, F. G., Barrera, M., & Martinez, C. R. (2004). The cultural adaptation of prevention interventions: Resolving tensions between fidelity and fit. *Society for Prevention Research*, Vol. 5, No. 1.

Chamberlin, J. (2005, April). 'A crucial time' for LGB research. *Monitor on Psychology*, 36(4), 84–85.

Chamberlin, J. (2006, June). It takes a community. *Monitor on Psychology*, 37(6), 24–25.

Depression Guideline Panel (1993). *Depression in primary care: Vol. 1, Diagnosis and detection* (Clinical Practice Guidelines No. 5, AHCPR Publication No. 93–0550). Rockville, MD: U.S. Department of Health and Human Services, Public Health Service, Agency for Health Care Policy and Research.

Dryman, A., & Eaton, W. W. (1991). Affected symptoms associated with the onset of major depression in the community: Findings from the U.S. National Institute of Mental Health Epidemiologic Catchment Area Program. *Acta Psychiatric Scandinavia*, 84, 1–5.

D'Zurilla, T. J., & Goldfried, M. R. (1971). Problem solving and behavior modification. *Journal of Abnormal Psychology*, 78(1), 107–126.

Epstein, S. (1967). Toward a unified theory of anxiety. In D. Mahar (Ed.), *Progress in experimental personality research* (Vol. 4, pp. 1–89). New York: Academic Press.

Farquhar, J. W., Fortman, S. P., Flora, J. A., Taylor, C. B. Haskell, W. L., Williams, P. T., et al. (1990). Effects of community wide education on cardiovascular disease risk factors: The Stanford Five City Project. *Journal of the American Medical Association*, 264, 359–365.

Feldman, R. A., & Wodarski, J. S. (1975). *Contemporary approaches to group treatment*. San Francisco, CA: Jossey-Bass.

Fischer, J. (1971). A framework for the analysis and comparison of clinical theories induced change. *Social Service Review*, 45(4), 440–454.

Fischer, J. (1978). *Effective case work practice*. New York: McGraw-Hill.

Forrest, J. D., & Singh, S. (1990). Public sector savings resulting from expenditures for contraceptive services. *Family Planning Perspectives*, 22(1), 6–15.

Gilchrist, L. D. (1981). Social confidence in adolescence. In S. Schinke (Ed.), *Behavioral methods in social welfare* (pp. 61–80). New York: Aldine.

Glaser, D. (1994). What works, and why it is important: A response to Logan and Gaes. *Justice Quarterly*, 11(4), 711–723.

Gold, M. R., Chu, R. C., Griffith, H. M., & Kamerow, D. B. (1993). *Preventive services in the clinical settings: What works and what it costs*. Washington, DC: Office of Disease Prevention and Health Promotion.

Goldstein, A. P., Sprafkin, R. P., Gershaw, N. J., & Klein, P. (1980). *Skill streaming the adolescent*. Champaign, IL: Research Press.

Greer, M. (2005, July/August). The protector. *Monitor on Psychology*, 36(7), 46.

Gross, A. M. (1980). Appropriate cost reporting: An indispensable link to accountability. *Administration in Social Work*, 4(3), 31–41.

Haggerty, R. J. (1977). *Relationship enhancement*. San Francisco, CA: Jossey-Bass.

Heller, K. (1996). Coming of age of prevention science: Comments on the 1994 National Institute of Mental Health-Institute of Medicine Prevention Reports. *American Psychologist*, 51(11), 1123–1127.

Henderson, A. S., Montgomery, I. M., & Williams, C. L. (1972). Psychological immunization: A proposal for preventive psychiatry. *Lancet*, 13, 1111–1112.

Hudson, W. W. (1982). *The clinical measurement package: A field manual*. Homewood, IL: Dorsey Press.

Kellam, S. G., & Rebok, G. W. (1992). Building developmental and etiological theory through epidemiologically based preventive intervention trials. In J. McCord & R. E. Tremblay (Eds.), *Preventing anti social behavior: Interventions from birth through adolescence* (pp. 162–198). New York: Guilford Press.

Kersting, K. (2005a, September). Suicide prevention efforts needed, American Indian psychologist tells policy-makers. *Monitor on Psychology*, 36(8), 12.

Kersting, K. (2005b, September). Caring for Medicaid. *Monitor on Psychology*, 36(8), 44.

Kessler, R. C., McGonale, K. A., Shauang, Z., Nelson, C. B., Hughes, M., Eshleman, S., et al. (1994). Lifetime and 12 month prevalence of DSM-III-R psychiatry disorders in the United States: Results from the National Comorbidity Survey. *Archives of General Psychiatry*, 51, 8–19.

Landsman, M. S. (1994). Needed: Metaphors for the prevention model of mental health. *American Psychologists*, 49(12), 1086–1087.

Lange, A. J., & Jakubowski, P. (1976). *Responsible assertiveness behavior*. Champaign, IL: Research Press.

Levin, H. M. (1983). *Cost effectiveness: A primer*. Newbury Park, CA: Sage.

Mahoney, M. J. (1974). *Cognition and behavior modification*. Cambridge, MA: Ballinger.

Marsiglio, W., & Mott, F. L. (1986). The impact of sex education on sexual activity, contraceptive use and premarital pregnancy among American teenagers. *Family Planning Perspective*, 18(4), 151–162.

McGinnis, J. M., & Foege, W. H. (1993). Actual causes of debt in the United States. *Journal of the American Medical Association*, 270, 2270–2212.

Meichenbaum, D. (1975). Self instructional methods. In F. Kanfer & A. Goldstein (Eds.), *Helping people change* (pp. 357–391). New York: Pergamon Press.

Meyer, R. G., & Smith, S. S. (1977). A crisis in group therapy. *American Psychologists*, 32, 638–643.

Mrazek, P. J., & Haggerty, R. J. (Eds.) (1994). *Reducing risk for mental disorders: Frontiers for preventive intervention research*. Washington, DC: National Academy Press.

National Center for Health Statistics (1990). *Health: United States 1990.* DHHA Pub. No. (PHS) 19–1232. Hyattsville, MD.

National Institute of Mental Health, Committee on Prevention Research (1995, May). *A plan for prevention research for the National Institute of Mental Health* (a report to the National Advisory Mental Health Council). Washington, DC: National Institute of Mental Health.

Perry, M. J., & Albee, G. W. (1994). On the signs of prevention. *American Psychologists,* 49, 1087–1088.

Rose, S. D. (1977). *Group therapy: A behavioral approach.* Englewood Cliffs, NJ: Prentice Hall.

Ross, H., & Glaser, E. (1973). Making it out of the ghetto. *Professional Psychology,* 4(3), 347–356.

Rusch, F. R. (Ed.) (1986). *Competitive employment issues and strategies.* Baltimore, MD: Paul H. Brooks.

Rusch, F. R. (1992). Identifying special education outcomes: Response to Ysseldyke, Thurlow, and Bruininks. *Remedial and Special Education,* 13(6), 31–32.

Schinke, S. P., & Gilchrist, L. D. (1984). *Life skills counseling with adolescents.* Baltimore, MD: University Park Press.

Schinke, S. P., Gilchrist, L. D., Smith, T. E., & Wong, S. E. (1979). Group interpersonal skills training in a natural setting: An experimental study. *Behavioral Research and Therapy,* 17, 149–154.

Schinke, S. P., & Rose, S. D. (1976). Interpersonal skills training in groups. *Journal of Counseling Psychology,* 23, 442–448.

Schoenborn, C. A., & Horn, J. (1993). *Negative moods as correlates of smoking and heavier drinking: Implications for health promotion.* Hyattsville, MD: National Center for Health Statistics.

Spivack, G., Platt, J. J., & Shure, M. B. (1976). *The problem solving approach to adjustment.* San Francisco, CA: Jossey-Bass.

Spivack, G., & Shure, M. B. (1974). *Social adjustment of young children.* San Francisco, CA: Jossey-Bass.

Stambor, Z. (2006, June). Prevention as intervention. *Monitor on Psychology,* 36(6), 30.

Stokey, E., & Zeckhauser, R. (1978). *A primer for policy analysis.* New York: W.W. Norton.

United States Bureau of the Census (1994). *Statistical abstracts of the United States* (114th ed.). Washington, DC: U.S. Government Printing Office.

United States General Accounting Office (1990). *Health insurance: Availability and adequacy for small businesses.* GAO/T-HRD-90–33. Washington, DC.

Weissberg, R. P., Kumpfer, K. L., & Seligman, M. E. P. (2003). Prevention that works for children and youth. *American Psychologist,* 58(6/7), 425–432.

Wells, K. B., Stewart, A., Hays, R. D., Burnam, M. A., Rogers, W., Daniels, M., et al. (1989). Detection of well being in depressed patients: Results from the Medical Outcomes Study. *Journal of the American Medical Association,* 262, 914–919.

Wodarski, L. A., Adelson, C. L., Todd, M. T., & Wodarski, J. S. (1980). Teaching nutrition by teams-games-tournaments. *Journal of Nutrition Education,* 12(2), 61–65.

Wodarski, J. S. (1981). *Role of research in clinical practice.* Austin, TX: PRO-ED.

Wodarski, J. S., & Bogarozzi, D. A. (1979). *Behavioral social work.* New York: Human Sciences Press.

Wodarski, J. S., & Feldman, R. A. (1973). The research practicum: A beginning formulation of process and educational objectives. *International Social Work*, 16(4), 42–48.

Wodarski, J. S., & Wodarski, L. A. (1993). *Curriculums and practical aspects of implementation: Preventive health services for adolescents.* Lanham, MD: University Press of America.

Wodarski, J. S., & Wodarski, L. A. (1998). *Adolescent violence: An empirically-based school/family paradigm.* New York: Springer.

Wodarski, J. S., Wodarski, L. A., & Parris, H. (2004). Teams—games—tournaments: Four decades of research. *Journal of Evidence-Based Social Work: Advances in Practice, Programming, Research and Policy*, 1(1), 23–43.

Summary

American Psychiatric Association (1994). *Diagnostic and statistical manual of mental disorders DSM-IV* (4th ed.). Washington, DC: American Psychological Association.

Arkava, M. L., & Brennen, E. C. (1975). Toward a competency examination for the baccalaureate social worker. *Journal of Education for Social Work*, 11(3), 22–29.

Armitage, A., & Clark, F. W. (1975). Design issues in the performance-based curriculum. *Journal of Education for Social Work*, 11(1), 22–29.

Backenstrab, M., Kronmuller K. T., Schwarz, T., Reck, C., Karr, M., Kocherscheidt, K. et al. (2001). Cognitive-behavioral psychotherapy with and within groups—A treatment program for depressed inpatients. *Verhaltenshtherapie*, 11(4), 305–311.

Baer B. L., & Federico, R. (1978). *Educating the baccalaureate social worker. Report of the undergraduate social work curriculum development project.* Cambridge, MA: Ballinger Publishing Company.

Bernstein, B. E. (1978, May). Points to ponder when seeking a new professional position. *Professional Psychology*, 9(2), 341–349.

Bock, R., & English, A. (1973). *Got me on the run.* Boston, MA: Beacon.

Brandon, J. S., & Folk, S. (1977). Runaway adolescents' perception of parents and self. *Adolescence*, 12(46), 175–187.

Breckler, S. J. (2005, April). Connecting to science. *Monitor on Psychology*, 36(4), 70.

Brennan, T., Huizinga, D., & Elliott, D. S. (1978). *The social psychology of runaways.* Lexington, MA: D.C. Heath.

Campbell, D. T. (1994). The social psychology of scientific validity: An epistemological perspective and a personalized history. In W. R. Shadish & S. Fuller (Eds.), *The social psychology of science* (pp. 124–161). New York: Guilford Press.

Christensen, A., Phillips, S., Glasgow, R. E., & Johnson, S. M. (1983). Parental characteristics and interactional dysfunction in families with child behavior problems: A preliminary investigation. *Journal of Abnormal Child Psychology*, 11, 153–166.

Collins, J. D. (1971). The effects of the conjugal relationship modification method on marital communication and adjustment. Unpublished doctoral dissertation, Pennsylvania State University.

Cowen, E., & Work, W. (1988). Resilient children, psychological wellness, and primary prevention. *American Journal of Community Psychology*, 16, 591–607.

Custer, G. (1994, November). Can universities be liable for incompetent grads? *APA Monitor*, 25(11), 7.

DeAngelis, T. (2005, May). Dynamic duos. *Monitor on Psychology*, 36(5), 36-39.

Dziegielewski, S. F., Wodarski, J. S., & Feit, M. (2005). Social service research: Efficacy, necessity and effectiveness. *Journal of Social Service Research*, 32(1), 1–16.

D'Zurilla, T. L., & Goldfried, M. R. (1971). Problem solving and behavior modification. *Journal of Abnormal Psychology*, 37, 107–126.

Ely, A. L., Guerney, G. G., & Stover, L. (1973). Efficacy of the training phase of conjugal therapy. *Psychotherapy: Theory, Research and Practice*, 10, 201–207.

Foos, J. A., Ottens, A. J., & Hill, L. K. (1991). Managed mental health: A primer for counselors. *Journal of Counseling and Development*, 69(4), 332–336.

Goldfried, M., & Goldfried A. (1975). Cognitive change methods. In F. Kanfer and A. Goldstein (Eds.), *Helping people change* (pp. 89–116). New York: Pergamon Press.

Greenberg M. T., Domitrovich, C., & Bumbarger, B. (2001, March). The prevention of mental disorders in school-aged children: Current state of the field. *Prevention & Treatment*, 4(1), 3–4.

Hepler, J., & Noble, J. (1990). Improving social work education: Taking responsibility at the door. *Social Work*, 35(2), 126–133.

Hildebrand, J. A. (1968). Reasons for runaways. *Crime and Delinquency*, 14, 42–48.

Himle, J. A., Rassi, S., Haghighatgou, H., Krone, K. P., Nesse, R. M., & Abelson, J. (2001). Group behavioral therapy of obsessive-compulsive disorder: Seven- vs. twelve-week outcomes. *Depression and Anxiety*, 13(4), 161–165.

Hoffman, M. L. (1977). Personality and social development. In M. R. Rosenzweig & L. W. Porter (Eds.), *Annual review of psychology* (Vol. 28, pp. 295–321). Palo Alto, CA: Annual Reviews.

Home, A., & Darveau-Fournier, L. (1982). A study of social work practice with groups. *Social Work with Groups*, 5(3), 19–34.

Houle, C. O., Cyphert, F., & Boggs, D. (1987, Spring). Education for the professions. *Theory into Practice*, 26(2), 87–93.

Howing, P. T., Hawkins, J. D., Lishner, D. M., Catalano, R. F., & Howard, M. O. (1986). Childhood predictions of adolescent substance abuse: Toward an empirically grounded theory. *Journal of Children in Contemporary Society*, 8, 11–48.

Johnson, A. A. (1975a, May). Community alternatives for adolescents. *Psychiatric Annals*, 5(5), 198–200.

Johnson, F. M. (1975b, September). Court decisions and the social services. *Social Work*, 20(5), 343–347.

Johnson, J. C. (1975c, September). The future of psychiatry in general hospitals. *Psychiatric Annals*, 5(9), 37–55.

Kersting, K. (2003, October). Bolstering evidence-based education. *Monitor on Psychology*, 34(9), 56–57.

Lederer, W., & Jackson, D. (1968). *The mirages of marriage*. New York: Norton.

Levant, R. F. (2005, February). Evidence-based practice in psychology. *Monitor on Psychology*, 36(2), 5.

Lochman, J. E. (2001, March). Prevention and treatment, issues in prevention with school-aged children: Ongoing intervention refinement, developmental theory, prediction and moderation, and implementation and dissemination. *Prevention & Treatment*, 4(1), 12–28. Electronic reference formats recommended by the Task Strategies: An Empirical Approach to Social Work Practice (1992). Retrieved on April 2, 2005, from http://www.taskcentered.com/empirica.htm.

Martin, R. (1974). *Behavior modification: Human rights and legal responsibilities*. Champaign, IL: Research Press.

Martin, R. (1975). *Legal challenges to behavior modification*. Champaign, IL: Research Press.

Morrison, N. (2001). Group cognitive therapy: Treatment of choice or sub-optimal option? *Behavioral and Cognitive Psychotherapy*, 29(3), 311–332.

NASW (2006). Code of ethics of the National Association of Social Workers. Retrieved July 21, 2006, from http://www.socialworkers.org/pubs/code/code.asp.

Parloff, M. B., Waskow, I. E., & Wolfe, B. E. (1978). Research on therapist variables in relation to process and outcome. In S. L. Garfield & A. E. Bergin (Eds.), *Handbook of psychotherapy and behavior change: An empirical analysis* (2nd ed., pp. 233–282). New York: Wiley.

Patterson, G. R., & Forgatch, M. S. (1987). *Parents and adolescents living together. Part 1: The basics*. Eugene, OR: Castalia.

Paul, G. L. (1969). Behavior modification research. In C. M. Franks (Ed.), *Behavior therapy: Appraisal and status* (pp. 29–62). New York, McGraw-Hill.

Randall, E., & Wodarski, J. S. (1989). Theoretical issues in clinical social group work. *Small Group Behavior*, 20(4), 475–499.

Rappaport, A., & Harrell, J. (1972). A behavioral exchange model for marital counseling. *The Family Coordinator*, 21, 203–212.

Reid, W. J. (1992). *Task strategies: An empirical approach to clinical social work*. New York: Columbia University Press.

Resnick, B. (1996a). Motivation in geriatric rehabilitation. *Journal of Nursing Scholarship*, 28(1), 41–45.

Resnick, M. (1996b). Toward a practice of "constructional design." In L. Schauble & R. Glaser (Eds.), *Innovations in learning: New environments for education* (pp. 161–174). Hillsdale, NJ: Lawrence Erlbaum Associates.

Rittner B., & Wodarski, J. S. (1995). Clinical assessment instruments in the treatment of child abuse and neglect. *Early Child Development and Care*, 106, 43–58.

Robin, A. L., & Foster, S. L. (1989). Negotiating parent-adolescent conflict: A behavioral family systems approach. *Behavior Therapist*, 13, 69.

Robinson, P. A. (1978). Parents of "beyond control" adolescents. *Adolescence*, 13, 109–119.

Sanderson, C. (1995a). *Counseling adult survivors of child sexual abuse* (2nd ed.). Philadelphia, PA: Jessica Kingsley Publishers.

Sanderson, J. (1995b). Helping families and professionals to work with children who have learning difficulties. In S. C. Smith & M. Pennells (Eds.), *Interventions with bereaved children* (pp. 219–231). Philadelphia, PA: Jessica Kingsley Publishers.

Satir, V. (1967). *Conjoint family therapy*. Palo Alto, CA: Basic Books.

Spivack G., & Shure, M. B. (1974). *Social adjustment of young children*. San Francisco, CA: Jossey-Bass.

Stein, H. D. (2003). *Challenge and change in social work education: Towards a world view: Observations and determinants of social work education in the United States* (pp. 62 & 80). Alexandria, Virginia: Council on Social Work Education.

Streever, K. L., Wodarski, J. S., & Lindsey, E. W. (1984). Assessing client change in human service agencies. *Family Therapy*, 11(2), 163–173.

Suddick, D. (1973). Runaways: A review of the literature. *Juvenile Justice*, 24, 46–54.

Thyer, B. A. (1995). Promoting an empiricist agenda within the human services: An ethical and humanistic imperative. *Journal of Behavior Therapy and Experimental Psychiatry*, 26(2), 93–98.

Thyer, B. A., & Wodarski, J. S. (2007). *Handbook of empirical social work practice, Vol. 2: Mental disorders*. New York: John Wiley & Sons.

Toseland, R. W., & Rivas, R. F. (2005). *An introduction to group work practice: The focus of group work practice* (pp. 4–15). Boston, MA: Pearson Education. Electronic reference formats recommended by the National Association of Social Workers (1999). Retrieved April 2, 2005, from http://www.socialworks.org/pubs/code.

Truax, C. B., & Carkhuff, R. R. (1967). *Toward effective counseling and psychotherapy: Training and practice.* Hawthorne, NY: Aldine Publishing Company.

U.S. Department of Health and Human Services (1991). *Healthy people 2000* (Publication No. 91–50212). Washington, DC: Government Printing Office.

U.S. Department of Health and Human Services (1995). *Healthy people 2000: Mid-course review and 1995 revisions.* Washington, DC: Government Printing Office.

Vanderloo, M. C. (1977). A study of coping behavior of runaway adolescents as related to situational stresses. *Dissertation Abstract International, 28,* 2387–2388B (University Microfilms No. 5–B).

Wodarski, J. S. (1976). Recent supreme court legal decisions: Implications for social work practice. Paper presented at the 103rd Annual Forum, National Conference on Social Welfare, Washington, DC.

Wodarski, J. S. (1981a, Fall). Discussion of "A critique of some of the newer treatment modalities." *Clinical Social Work Journal, 9*(3), 171–176.

Wodarski, J. S. (1981b, Winter). Comprehensive treatment of parents who abuse their children. *Adolescence, 16*(64), 959–972.

Wodarski, J. S. (1985). *Introduction to human behavior.* Austin, TX: PRO-ED.

Wodarski, J. S. (2000). The role for social workers in the managed health care system: A model for empirically based psycho-social interventions. *Crisis intervention and time limited treatment, 6*(2), 109–139.

Wodarski, J. S., Feit, M. D., & Green, R. K. (1995). Graduate social work education: A review of two decades of empirical research and considerations for the future. *Social Service Review, 69(1),* 108–130.

Wodarski, J. S., & Hilarski, C. (in press). *Handbook of evidence based social work education.* Binghamton, NY: Haworth Press.

Wodarski, J. S., & Thyer, B. A. (1989). Behavioral perspectives on the family: An overview. In B. Thyer (Ed.), *Behavioral family interventions.* Springfield, IL: Charles C. Thomas.

Wodarski, J. S., & Wodarski, L. A. (1993). *Curriculums and practical aspects of implementation: Preventive health services for adolescents.* Lanham, MD: University Press of America.

Yalom, I. D. (1995). *The theory and practice of group psychotherapy* (4th ed.). New York: Basic Books.

Index

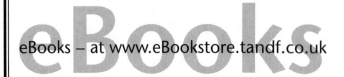